CRANIOSACRAL THERAPY II
Beyond the Dura

CRANIOSACRAL THERAPY II
Beyond the Dura

John E. Upledger
D.O., F.A.A.O.

Illustrations by
LILIAN LAI BENSKY

Eastland Press
SEATTLE

Book design by Catherine L. Nelson.
Photolithoprinted by Cushing-Malloy, Incorporated,
Ann Arbor, Michigan, 1987.

Fourth Printing, 1992

This book is dedicated to all of you, the students of craniosacral therapy, who have been so supportive and understanding as we suffered the trials and tribulations which accompanied the release of this work to the public. We have done this so that health care practitioners from all disciplines can learn it if they desire, and so that a much larger segment of the population may benefit from it.

Thank you.

TABLE OF CONTENTS

ACKNOWLEDGMENTS

Thank you, Dianne Upledger, for putting up with me as I wrote and cursed and researched and referenced and loved every minute of this work. Thank you, Geri Foltz and Nancy Royster, for translating my handwritten hieroglyphics into a legible and meaningful typewritten manuscript. Thank you, Dan Bensky, John O'Connor and Steve Anderson, editors of Eastland Press, for keeping me honest and at times offering criticism or pointing out error.

I would also like to thank all of the people who have created the Upledger Institute. Their faith and dedication have been of inestimable value.

PREFACE

This book is an extension of my first book on the subject, *Craniosacral Therapy* (UPLEDGER 1983). It extends deeper into the known body of anatomical knowledge. It also extends further into the unknown. I am sure it will stimulate more discussion and controversy among its readers.

My objectives in chapter 1 are to broaden your scope of knowledge and understanding of the cranial nerves and how they can be effectively influenced by craniosacral therapy. I have also attempted to integrate the peripheral cranial nerve systems individually with their central nervous system (brain) connections, and thus begin to clarify how some craniosacral system dysfunctions can have such a dramatic impact on total behavior. Many questions, as yet unanswered, arise from this probing.

In chapter 2, I have also tried to verbally and pictorially dissect the fascial anatomy of the neck, and to bring it into focus from a craniosacral point of view. Of course, in order to perform this fascial dissection, we have to consider in detail the structures to which these fasciae attach. I do hope that this description will simplify a rather complex area of the human body. My goal is to provide a reasonably simple model of cervical soft tissue anatomy with which you can effectively understand and facilitate the correction of all types of cervical function problems.

The temporomandibular joint is scrutinized in chapter 3. I am sure that I have stepped on some toes in this part of the book, but controversy is healthy. If we knew all about the "TMJ syndrome," there would be no disagreement. My purpose in this section is to present a craniosacrally oriented view of the functional anatomy of the temporomandibular joint. I have tried to place the anatomy of the joint in the context of the whole person, and then to consider what we as therapists can do to aid the "TMJ syndrome" sufferer.

In chapter 4, I discuss concepts and observations which have unfolded for me since writing *Craniosacral Therapy*. I have very little scientific evidence to support most of these observations. However, these are phenomena that I have personally observed, and I have attempted to describe only what I have seen. My goal in doing so is to pique the reader's curiosity, and perhaps widen your vision so that the depth of your comprehension of the wonders of the human organism may increase as mine has.

Please enjoy the book, use it as a reference and as a stimulation to your thought. If you see things that you want to share with me, I would appreciate your doing just that. I do have more work than I can handle, but I love sharing new ideas and observations. I'll try hard to answer your letter.

John E. Upledger, D.O., F.A.A.O.
Palm Beach Gardens, Florida

1.

CRANIAL NERVES

CHAPTER 1

I. INTRODUCTION

The cranial nerves are frequently regarded as being twelve pair of peripheral nerves which relate to the sensory and motor activities of the head. It is not strictly correct, however, to regard the olfactory and optic nerves (cranial nerves I and II, respectively) as peripheral nerves. They are actually peripheral extensions of brain fiber tracts because there is no synapse between their sensory end organs and entries into the substance of the brain. Despite this misnomer and in order to avoid further confusion, our discussion will bow to the traditional nomenclature and refer to them as being among the twelve pair of cranial nerves.

Cranial nerves III through XII, on the other hand, are true peripheral nerves because they synapse external to the central nervous system. These ten pair of cranial nerves all have their superficial entries and exits to and from the brain stem. All have their nuclei within the brain stem as well, except the spinal accessory nerve (XI) which has a part of its nucleus in the upper and middle cervical spinal cord. This nucleus is known accordingly as the spinal nucleus of the accessory nerve.

In addition to the head, the cranial nerves also have significant functions in the neck, thorax and abdomen. The glossopharyngeal nerve (IX) supplies both sensory and motor fibers to the pharynx and larynx, both of which extend into the neck. The vagus nerve (X) innervates the organs of the digestive, circulatory and respiratory systems in addition to its functions in the head. The accessory nerve supplies motor innervation to the pharynx and larynx as well as the sternocleidomastoid and trapezius muscles of the neck.

The cranial nerves are often viewed erroneously as the cranial part of the parasympathetic division of the autonomic nervous system. This is probably because the parasympathetic division is sometimes called the craniosacral division of the autonomic nervous system. Although several parasympathetic fibers "hitch a ride" with the cranial nerves, that's about all there is to it. The cranial nerves contain an abundance of peripheral sensory fibers. All of these sensory fibers have their cells of origin external to the brain stem, usually from ganglia which might be considered analogous to the dorsal root ganglia of the spinal cord. The cranial nerves also contain voluntary peripheral motor fibers which innervate structures of the musculoskeletal and myofascial systems. Clearly, the cranial nerves are very heterogeneous in their composition, containing parasympathetic fibers as well as peripheral sensory and voluntary motor fibers.

A specific nerve trunk may be thought of as a transportation route which offers a convenient means of travel for specialized nerve fibers from one region of the body to another. In most cases, fibers from the common trunk carry out many different, individualized or specialized functions. This is not always the case, however, as some nerve trunks carry only one type of fiber for one specific purpose. An example of singular function would be the trochlear nerve (IV). As far as we know at present, this nerve contains only motor fibers which innervate the superior oblique muscle of the eye.

The important point to keep in mind is that, more often than not, the peripheral nerve is a convenient means of routing specialized nerve fibers with very diverse functions from one region of the body to another. As a major nerve trunk passes through an area of specific assignment for a motor fiber tract, the specialized fibers exit the nerve trunk as a branch, while the trunk continues to its more peripheral destination. I use the word "exit" to describe the "branching" of motor nerves. In the case of sensory input, we might consider the sensory afferent fibers as "tributaries" which "enter" the nerve trunk as a means of moving impulses in a central direction.

The decision as to which fibers join which nerves is determined by the origin and destination of the nerve impulse. An analogy might be a routing schedule of a trip from Chicago to Los Angeles for a truck moving several households of furniture on the same trip, loading and unloading at specific places. With this concept in mind, many of the more baffling syndromes and dysfunctions which arise from mechanical deformations and/or deteriorative processes of specific nerves in specific anatomical locations become easier to understand.

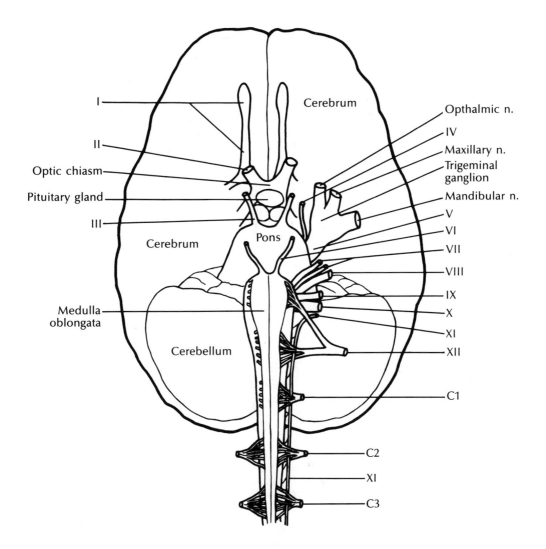

Illustration 1-1
Cranial Nerves Viewed From Underside of the Brain

I have come to regard the cranial nerves as being similar to the spinal nerves in terms of their arrangement as they exit and enter the brainstem. The similarity is apparent if you look at the spinal cord as a caudal extension of the brainstem. In general, you can think in terms of "brainstem segments" with cranial nerves as segmental nerve roots. This provides a convenient way of organizing what superficially appears to be a very complex system (ILLUSTRATION 1-1). To carry this analogy a step further, you can then think of the jugular foramina as intervertebral foramina between the occiput and the sphenoid. These foramina allow passage of cranial nerves IX, X and XI just as the spinal nerve roots pass through the intervertebral foramina below (ILLUSTRATION 1-2). As we discuss the functional and dysfunctional anatomy of the various cranial nerves the usefulness of this model will become apparent.

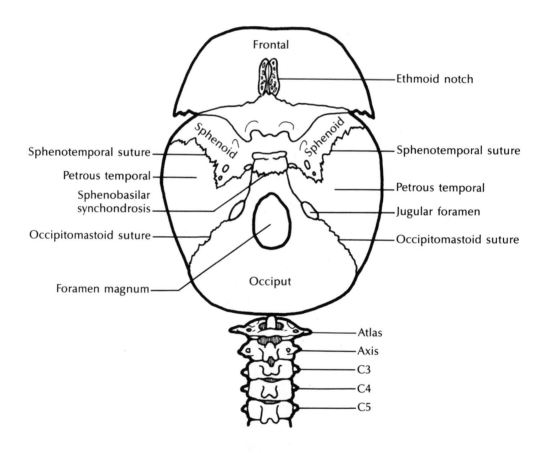

Illustration 1-2
Analogy of Jugular Foramina to
Intervertebral Foramina

The cranial nerves are the following:

    I Olfactory (special sensory)
   II Optic (special sensory)

   III   Oculomotor (somatic and visceral motor)
   IV   Trochlear (somatic motor)
    V   Trigeminal (somatic sensory and somatic motor)
   VI   Abducens (somatic motor)
  VII   Facial (somatic and visceral sensory/motor)
 VIII   Vestibulocochlear [auditory or acoustic] (special sensory)
   IX   Glossopharyngeal (somatic and visceral sensory/motor)
    X   Vagus (somatic and visceral sensory/motor)
   XI   Accessory (somatic motor; assists vagus)
  XII   Hypoglossal (somatic motor)

Let us now consider each of the cranial nerves and their systems in terms of function, dysfunctional manifestations and vulnerabilities.

II. OLFACTORY SYSTEM

A. General anatomy

The olfactory nerve (I) is not a true peripheral nerve. It is a fiber tract of the brain which enters into the inferior surface of the frontal lobe. The paired olfactory nerves arise from sensory receptors located in the nasal mucosa (mucous membranes) of the superior nasal cavities. There are about 20 non-myelinated fibers on each side which pass from these sensory receptors up through the tiny foramina in the cribriform plate of the ethmoid bone to the olfactory bulbs of the brain (ILLUSTRATION 1-3). The cribriform plates fit into the ethmoid notch of the frontal bone between the two orbits of the eyes (ILLUSTRATION 1-4).

After entering the substance of the brain at the olfactory bulbs, these sensory fibers have their first synaptic juncture. The unmyelinated fibers, which have ascended from the mucous membranes of the nasal cavities, have synapses with myelinated fibers of the olfactory tracts of the frontal lobes of the brain. These olfactory tracts then travel posteriorly through the substance of the brain to the subcallosal and hippocampal gyri. Here there is another synaptic juncture with fibers going to the pyriform and hippocampal areas of the brain. These connections are made via the medial and lateral olfactory stria.

Associated fibers connect these areas with the tegmentum, the pons and the thalamus. Reflex connections are also present which provide communication between the olfactory system and the nuclei of the trigeminal (V), glossopharyngeal (IX), vagus (X) and hypoglossal (XII) nerves (ILLUSTRATION 1-5).

B. Function and dysfunction

What does all this anatomy mean? When an odor (consisting of tiny chemical particles, molecules or ions) reaches the roof of the nasal cavities, the sensory receptors in the nasal mucosa convert the chemical stimulation into nerve impulses. In order for the sensory receptors to respond to the odor, the chemical must be dissolved in

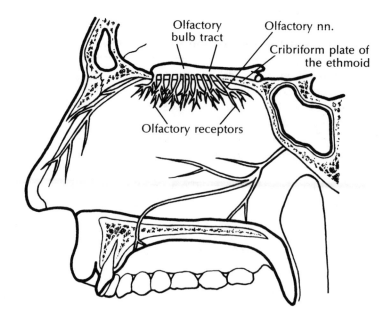

Illustration 1-3
Passage of Olfactory Nerves Through Cribriform Plate

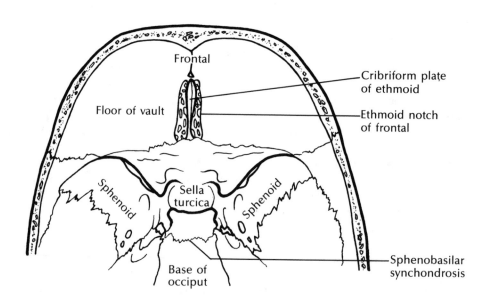

Illustration 1-4
Anterior Cranial Fossa Including Cribriform Plate

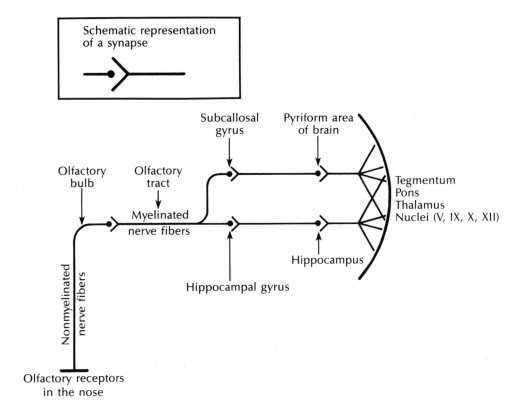

Illustration 1-5
Schematic Representation of the Olfactory System

the fluid which the mucous membranes secrete. Without the particles going into solution, the receptors are not activated. A common cause of loss of smell (which is called olfactory desensitization) is dry nose. Perhaps you have noticed some loss of the acuteness of your sense of smell when you are in a very dry climate or when you are using medicinal agents which dry up the nasal mucous membranes. Of course, the nose also must be open so that odor particles can reach the upper nasal cavities. When you have a severe cold with rhinitis (runny nose) and swelling of the turbinates, access to the olfactory sensory areas is limited and the sense of smell is also reduced.

As the sensory fibers ascend from the nasal cavity in bundles, each bundle is ensheathed by dura mater and pia mater membranes. The dural membranes are continuous with the periosteum of the nasal bones, and the pial membranes are continuous with the perineurium of the fiber tract bundles. This relationship with the dural membrane is a possible source of interference with the transmission of impulses from the olfactory sensory receptors to the brain. The dural membrane must be supple, otherwise it may cause mechanical deformation and abnormal tension upon the bundles of the olfactory nerve. The sense of smell may then be compromised.

The dural membrane is attached to the ethmoid and frontal bones. Therefore, mechanical interference with the free mobility of either of these two bones may result in abnormal dural tension and secondary problems with the sense of smell.

Trauma to the nose which causes undue tension upon the dural sheaths can also interfere with the sense of smell. Since the dura mater becomes the periosteum of the nasal bones, it is easy to see how a post-traumatic malposition of these bones can cause abnormal dural tension.

1. Ethmoid. One must likewise consider the effects of dysfunction of the vomer, ethmoid, frontal and sphenoid bones in cases of olfactory impairment. Olfactory receptor cells are located on the superior concha and on the upper septum of the ethmoid bone. The olfactory nerve bundles must pass without interference through the tiny holes in the cribriform plate of the ethmoid. The olfactory bulbs lie on the superior surface of the ethmoid lateral to the crista galli. Normal ethmoid function is essential to a normal sense of smell.

The ethmoid is most vulnerable to dysfunction secondary to problems with the frontal, vomer or sphenoid bones (ILLUSTRATION 1-6).

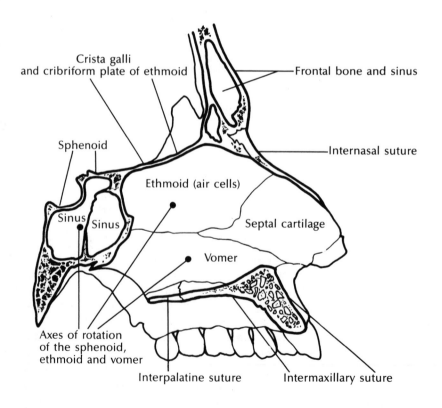

Crista galli
and cribriform plate of ethmoid — Frontal bone and sinus

Sphenoid

Internasal suture

Ethmoid (air cells)

Sinus Sinus

Septal cartilage

Vomer

Axes of rotation
of the sphenoid,
ethmoid and vomer

Interpalatine suture   Intermaxillary suture

Illustration 1-6
Midsagittal View of the Bony Structures
Affecting the Olfactory Nerve

The ethmoid bone is subject to lateral pressure from the frontal, as well as immobility due to frontal flexion, extension, torsioning or compression. Further, the frontal is very much at the mercy of abnormal tensions on the falx cerebri, which may be coming from almost anywhere along the vertical membrane system (UPLEDGER 1983, CHAPTER 6).

2. Vomer. The vomer is driven largely by the sphenoid. It has an extensive articulation with the ethmoid adjacent to and in front of its articulation with the sphenoid. The vomer-sphenoid articulation is a tongue and groove design which well serves its purpose, but which also makes it extremely vulnerable to compressive jamming. I have seen many cases wherein facial trauma resulted in jamming of this joint (ILLUSTRATION 1-7).

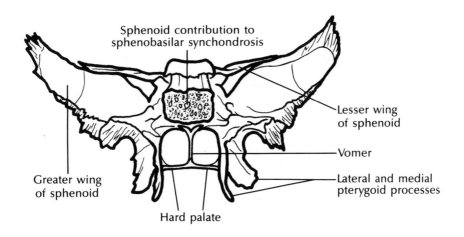

Illustration 1-7
Posterior View of the Sphenoid, Vomer
and Hard Palate

Further vomer vulnerability is seen in its articular relationships to the hard palate. This is another long and intricate tongue and groove joint which may also become jammed (though less frequently than the vomer-sphenoid joint), resulting in impaired free motion of the vomer (ILLUSTRATION 1-8).

3. Sphenoid. Because it is driven so powerfully by its direct connection to the craniosacral hydraulic system, the sphenoid is not often motion-restricted to the extent that it impairs ethmoidal function. The ethmoid has little if any mechanically significant and direct connection with the hydraulic aspect of the craniosacral system, except via the anterior falx cerebri attachment to the cribriform plate. Sphenoid-caused ethmoidal dysfunction is actually not rare, but it occurs less often than ethmoidal dysfunction secondary to frontal and/or vomeral restriction. Sphenoidal restriction can occur for many reasons. In my own experience, it is the severe anterior-posterior compression of the sphenoid with the occiput that most often causes ethmoidal dysfunction with secondary impairment of the olfactory system.

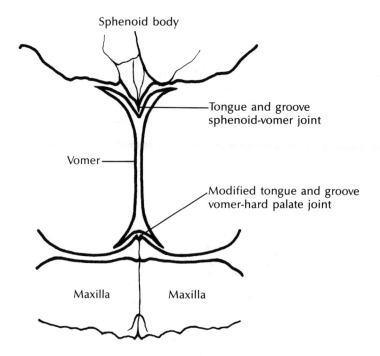

Illustration 1-8
Posterior Close-up View of the Vomer's
Articulation with the Sphenoid and Hard Palate

4. Summary. So, between the olfactory sensory receptors of the nose and the entry of the olfactory fibers into the brain substance we see potential for problems in several areas:

- Obstruction of nasal passages
- Abnormally dry or wet nasal passages
- Abnormal dural membrane tension affecting the fibers of the olfactory nerve
- Bony dysfunction, either directly affecting the olfactory fibers or creating abnormally increased dural membrane tension

As we consider the connections of the olfactory system with other brain centers, we can begin to appreciate how Nature has designed this circuitry so that our sensory input and our actions are well integrated. It is well-known that smell lends a great deal to the sensation of taste. In fact it is almost impossible to tell, subjectively, which of our general impressions of flavor come from the tongue and which come from the nose.

C. Relationship to other areas of the brain

There are numerous interrelationships between the olfactory system and the nuclei of the trigeminal, glossopharyngeal, vagus and hypoglossal nerves. These intercommunications contribute significantly to the integration between the senses of taste and smell and the digestive functions. Consider that just the smell of onions cooking can make your mouth water and the stomach acids begin to flow. It is certain that nasal congestion and obstruction due to a cold can render food tasteless (or is it odorless?). The limbic system and the triune model of the brain are of particular interest in this context. They will be described in some detail.

1. Limbic system. The limbic system of the brain is sometimes referred to as the "mammalian brain," in contrast to the brainstem, or "reptilian brain." The limbic system may be envisioned as a V-shaped structure sitting on top of the brainstem and below the diencephalon, with the apex of the V pointing anteriorly. The word limbus in Latin means border.

The limbic system includes the amygdala, hippocampus, cingulum, septal nuclei (which protrude into the lateral ventricles from the medial side), part of the thalamus (hobenular nucleus and the rostral thalamic nucleus), parts of the hypothalamus (the mammillary bodies) and the intercrural nucleus of the mesencephalon (which connects to the reticular formation of the brainstem and ultimately to the visceral motor columns). Also included in the limbic system are many interconnecting neural pathways (ILLUSTRATION 1-9).

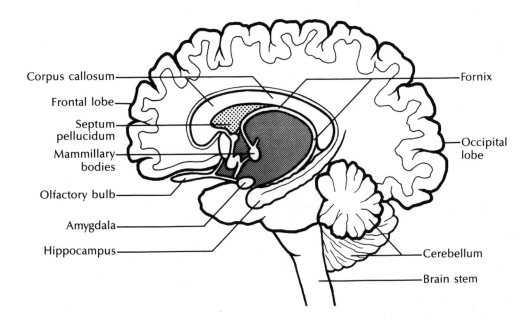

Illustration 1-9
The Limbic System

The limbic system receives sensory input from the olfactory, visual, auditory, balance and equilibrium systems, and from muscle proprioceptors; it seems to process much of this input and channel it in proper directions to the cortex and to the reticular activating system. The limbic system has multiple connections with the thalamus, hypothalamus and pituitary gland.

Functionally, the limbic system is the major seat of emotions. These emotions range from love and altruism to rage and panic. The anteriorly situated apex of the system is in the olfactory cortex, which explains the close relationship between smells and emotions. The limbic system has such generous connections with the sense of smell that it used to be called the rhinencephalon ("nose brain"). The olfactory cortex is the oldest part of the limbic system in terms of its evolution. In humans the limbic system is located behind and slightly above the nostrils. Most mammals are powerfully influenced by olfactory stimuli. Humans have not lost this connection, although visual stimuli have assumed greater importance than olfactory stimuli in terms of behavioral responses.

Within the brain substance the olfactory system connects extensively with the limbic system, which comprises about 20% of total brain volume. In view of the olfactory-limbic system connections, it is small wonder that the perfume business has done so well. It is very possible that certain smells arouse romantic or sentimental feelings in us.

The hippocampus is a paired organ. One is located in each temporal lobe of the brain. The hippocampus is involved in memory function. Its normal function depends upon a balance between the neurotransmitter substances GABA (gamma amino butyric acid) and glutamate (RESTAK 1984). Hippocampal areas are quite vulnerable to anoxia during the birth process. The resultant hippocampal damage usually causes seizures and memory disorder. In relationship to the olfactory system, the hippocampus helps us to remember such things as familiar fragrances. As we sense or perceive an odor from the olfactory system, the hippocampus compares that odor to its "memory bank" to determine whether it is a familiar fragrance, and if so, which related memories should be ushered forth into our conscious awareness.

The amygdala (paired) are located bilaterally in the limbic system just above the hypothalamus in the anterior tip of the temporal lobes. It is here that stimulation may create a rage-aggression response. It is thought that the amygdala works with the hypothalamus to mediate emotional responses. In many mammals, certain odors (probably hormonal) sensed by the olfactory system can precipitate rage and aggression. Such responses are not usually noticeable in humans, but the instinct may still be present in a vestigial form.

The septum pellucidum seems to be a pleasure center. Artificial electrical stimulation has produced happiness in depressed persons, pain relief in cancer victims and intensification of sexual arousal in normal people. Dysfunction of the septum can disrupt the ability to experience pleasure.

Limbic connections with the brain stem below, and the cerebrum above, allow for a balance and integration among alertness, emotion and reason. Consider the significance of the olfactory input into this limbic system. What might sensory (olfactory) deprivation do to the function of the limbic system and its mediatory function among alertness, emotion and reason?

2. Triune brain. The triune model of the brain was developed by Paul D. MacLean, formerly chief of the National Institute of Mental Health Laboratory for Brain Evolution. The model hypothesizes three separate but intimately related brains in humans, reflecting the phylogenetic stages of human evolution (RESTAK 1984, SAGAN 1977, WONDER 1984). The most primitive brain is the reptilian brain (or R-complex), which includes the spinal cord, medulla and pons. This brain is responsible for survival instincts and behavior necessary for self-preservation and propagation of the species. The instincts for hunting, mating, staking out territory and fighting for survival and the protection of territory are governed by the R-complex. It also conducts information into, and carries out orders from the neocortex.

Layered on top of the brainstem, like a cap, is the limbic system. Above the limbic system is the more highly-evolved cerebral cortex (ILLUSTRATION 1-10).

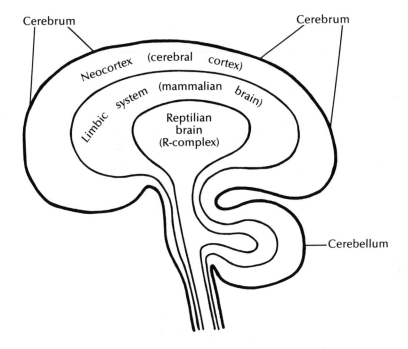

Illustration 1-10
Triune Model of the Brain

I find it interesting that nature sees fit to cap each brain structure with a more evolved brain, rather than to replace one with another. Each cap modifies and acts to control or inhibit the innate drives and instincts of the caps which are under or central to it. However, the influence or energy of each of the two caps beneath the neocortex is still present. Witness the evolutionary regression of human behavior under the influence of alcohol, which interferes with neocortical function first. When neocortical activity is inhibited, the capacity for abstract reasoning begins to disappear. We see the sentimental, loyal, emotional drunk. If the mammalian brain is then impaired we see the feisty, territorial drunk who says you better get out of his way and who is far beyond reason. When the R-complex becomes impaired, we see the primitive physiological control centers of the brainstem laboring to keep the drunk breathing and alive.

3. Reticular formation. This system is composed of several million neurons which form a dense network of fibers located mainly within the brainstem (or, in terms of the triune model, R-complex). The reticular formation extends from the thalamus through the midbrain, the pons and the medulla and down the spinal cord all the way to its sacral end. It is centrally located as it passes through the brainstem and spinal cord.

This formation comprises the major component of the nervous system in primitive vertebrates, and retains functional importance in birds and mammals (including humans). Stimulation of the reticular formation activates the reticular alarm system; overstimulation results in hyper-alertness. Destruction of the formation results in coma and death.

The system receives and processes millions of sensory messages daily. It prioritizes the information, acts on it when appropriate and serves as a triage officer relaying the input messages to the appropriate areas of the cerebral cortex for information, further decision making and action. The information which comes into the reticular formation has largely to do with visual light, taste and smell, as opposed to proprioceptive and discriminatory touch sensations.

The reticular formation alerts you to a dangerous smell, a bad taste, a visual danger signal, etc. It is the system that perks up a dog's ears when an odor wafts past from a nearby cat or other animal. It is integral to the arousal-sleep cycles of living things, and "decides" what is worth arousing you from sleep for.

The formation contains centers for the control of blood pressure, heart rate and respiratory rate. It has intimate interconnections with the trigeminal system, the optic system and the facial and glossopharyngeal systems (insofar as the latter two are concerned with taste).

4. Other connections. The olfactory system is connected to the thalamus, an egg-shaped mass located just above the brain stem. The thalamus also has abundant neural connections with the limbic system and acts as a relay station between sensory and motor nerves and the brain. Via the hypothalamus, the thalamus also functionally connects with the pituitary gland. Thus, there is a pathway whereby olfactory sensory stimuli can influence endocrine function.

The olfactory system provides sensory input to the pons, which is located at the front of the brainstem above the medulla. The pons provides interconnections between the cerebrum and the two hemispheres of the cerebellum; it is believed to be involved in control of respiration, REM sleep and the onset of dreaming (ILLUSTRATION 1-11).

The olfactory system has connections with the piriform lobe (collectively the lateral olfactory stria, anterior part of the parahippocampal gyrus and the uncus) and the tegmentum, which is part of the paleoencephalon ("old brain") which governs primitive responses and sensations related to metabolism and reproduction (e.g., hunger, thirst, fatigue and sex).

Research on the role of the olfactory system in overall brain function and human behavior is in its early stages. If one accepts the concept that sensory stimulation enhances developmental function of nerve tissue, and conversely that sensory deprivation results in reduction of nerve function and development, the possible implications of anosmia for the emotional life of a patient can readily be imagined.

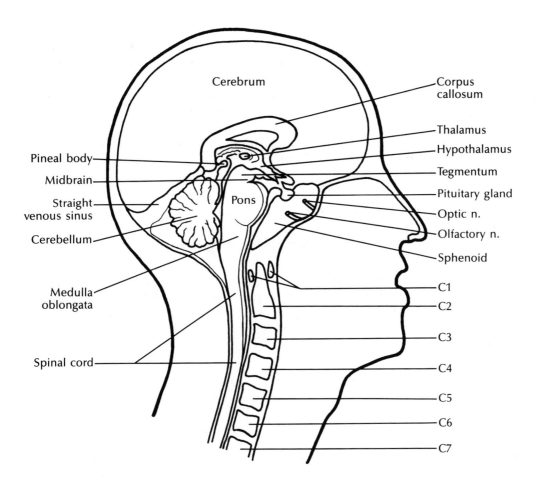

Illustration 1-11
Midsagittal View of Midbrain and Brainstem

III. VISUAL SYSTEM

A. Sensory input

1. Photoreceptors. The optic nerve (II) is primarily sensory (BUT SEE SECTION III.A.4), and involved in visual perception. Like the olfactory nerve, it is more correctly regarded as a fiber tract extension of the brain tissue rather than a peripheral nerve; there is no synapse between its sensory receptors in the retina and its axonic entry into the brain.

Stimulus to this nerve is by light entering the eye. Components of the retina convert light energy to electrical impulses which are conducted by the optic nerves, via the thalamus, to the visual cortex located bilaterally on the occipital lobes of the cerebrum. Integration and interpretation of the sensory information takes place in the visual cortex.

The photoreceptors (called rods and cones) which convert light energy to nerve impulses are, surprisingly, located on the inner layer of the retina; light must pass through several layers of other tissues to reach them. Each retina contains approximately 125 million rods and 7 million cones. These two types of photoreceptors are responsible for light/dark and color perception, respectively. They contain molecules (called visual pigments) whose structure is altered by contact with photons. The visual pigment of the rods is called rhodopsin, or visual purple. Exposure to light splits rhodopsin into retinene and opsin; this chemical reaction is accompanied by release of energy which stimulates the optic nerve.

There are three types of cone photoreceptors, each with a different visual pigment responding to a different light wave length (red, green and blue). The broad range of colors which we perceive is based on stimulation of these three cone types in varying proportions depending on the wave length composition of the light entering our eyes. Again, there is a chemical reaction in cone receptors which converts light energy to electrical energy and stimulates the optic nerve.

Cones are much less sensitive to dim light than are rods. This is why less intense colored light stimuli reaching the retina are perceived as less colorful, even as shades of gray. There is also little color perception in our peripheral vision because the cones are concentrated in one central area (the fovea centralis) on the retina; the rods are more widely distributed.

2. Retina/optic disk. Within each eyeball are over one million nerve cell bodies, the axons of which converge onto the optic disk located in the stratum opticum (nerve fiber) layer of the retina about 3mm medial to the posterior pole of the eyeball. From the optic disk, the axons exit the eyeball by passing through the choroid and scleral coverings. The sclera is the tough outer coating of the eyeball. It is about 0.8mm thick posteriorly. The axons pass through many tiny foramina (lamina cribrosa) in the sclera and join together posteriorly to the eyeball to form the optic nerve, at which point they become myelinated (ILLUSTRATION 1-12).

The optic disk is the blind spot of the eye; there are no photoreceptors on the disk itself. Since the two blind spots are medial to the posterior poles of the eyeballs, light waves from a single external point do not strike both blind spots at once. When light waves from an outside point do fall on a blind spot, we lose the image in that eye only. For this reason, because the optic disk covers only a small fraction of the retinal surface, and because the eyes are almost constantly moving, we seldom lose our stereoscopic perception of outside objects.

About 1.25cm posterior to the optic disk, the central retinal artery, which has been running anteriorly in the dural sheath of the optic nerve, pierces the nerve and enters the eyeball (ILLUSTRATION 1-13). This is the artery which is clearly seen with the ophthalmoscope in the center of the optic disk. It is a branch of the ophthalmic artery (a branch of the internal carotid artery which enters the bony orbit through the optic foramen).

There is a sheath of dura mater which envelops the optic nerve between its exit from the eyeball and its passage through the optic foramen, located in the lesser wing of the sphenoid (ILLUSTRATION 1-14). This sheath blends with the sclera and attaches to the superior osseous margin of the optic foramen.

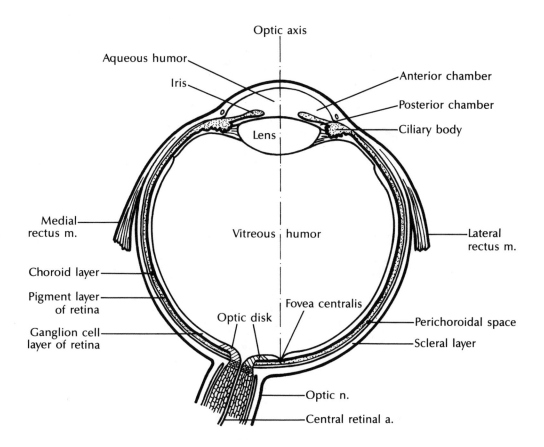

Illustration 1-12
Transverse Section of the Eyeball

3. Optic nerve. Within the orbit, the optic nerve is invested by sheaths which are continuous with all three meningeal layers of the cranial vault. The external surface of the orbit is considered to be outside of the cranial vault by virtue of its continuity with the external surface of the skull. The dura mater, arachnoid and pia mater all fuse with the sclera at the lamina cribrosa on the posterior eyeball.

As the ensheathed optic nerve passes from the sclera to the optic foramen, it is surrounded by a layer of fascia (called the fascia bulbi because it encapsulates the eyeball and allows movement relative to the sclera), an orbital fat pad and (anteriorly) ciliary arteries and nerves. Posteriorly, but still within the orbit, it is crossed over by the nasociliary nerve, ophthalmic artery, superior ophthalmic vein and superior division of the oculomotor nerve. The inferior division of the oculomotor nerve and the inferior rectus muscle of the eyeball pass underneath the optic nerve; the medial rectus muscle passes medial to it; and the lateral rectus muscle and abducens nerve pass lateral to it.

In the posterior extreme of the orbit, the optic nerve is in close approximation to the ciliary ganglion and the ophthalmic artery (from which it receives vascular branches). The distance the optic nerve travels from the sclera to the optic foramen

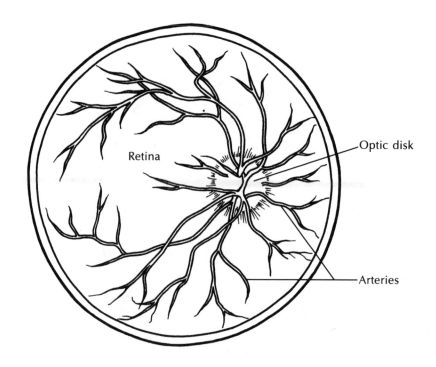

Illustration 1-13
Opthalmoscopic View of the Retina

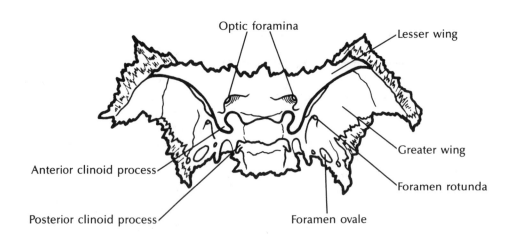

Illustration 1-14
Superior Aspect of the Sphenoid
and Optic Foramina

is about 2.5cm. There is some laxity of tension in the nerve to allow for movement of the eyeball.

As the optic nerve passes through the optic foramen, which is 5-10mm long, it passes over the top of the ophthalmic artery just after it has branched from the internal carotid. On its medial side, the optic nerve is separated from the sphenoid air sinuses by a very thin lamina of bone. In some cases, when the content of the air sinus cells (of the ethmoid as well as the sphenoid) is great, the nerve may be subject to pressure from all sides, with resulting visual disturbances. Variability of the air sinus cells may be due to inflammation of their mucoperiosteal linings.

As the nerve passes through the foramen, the three sheaths fuse to each other, to the periosteum of the bone and to the nerve itself. This fusion occurs only superiorly. This arrangement fixes the nerve in place so that it will not slide in and out of the orbit too freely. The separation between the meningeal layers is maintained in the inferior two-thirds of the sheath (ILLUSTRATION 1-15). The fixation of the nerve to the sphenoid in this manner subjects the function of the nerve to the influence of the bone, its sinuses and the closely-related ethmoid sinuses.

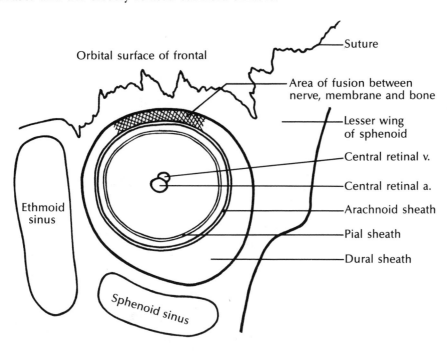

Illustration 1-15
Some of the Structures Which Affect
Eyeball Function

The intracranial portion of the nerve rests upon the superior surface of the cavernous venous sinus, and on the diaphragma sellae which overlies the pituitary gland. The third ventricle is close above. Laterally, the internal carotid is in close approximation; the ophthalmic branch is given off directly below the nerve. The anterior cerebral artery crosses above the nerve just before the nerve forms the optic chiasm (the junction with the contralateral nerve). Pressure on the nerve from aneurysm of any of these large arteries may present very early as visual system dysfunction.

4. Optic chiasm/optic tracts. The two optic nerves form the optic chiasm just above the diaphragma sellae (ILLUSTRATION 1-16). Thus, enlargement of the pituitary gland can also present as visual dysfunction. Sensory axons from the medial retinal fields (corresponding to the lateral visual fields) cross within the optic chiasm; those from the lateral retinal fields (corresponding to the medial or central visual field) do not cross, but continue to the ipsilateral visual cortex. Thus, pressure on the optic chiasm from an enlarged pituitary gland may present as loss of lateral visual field perception, or "tunnel vision."

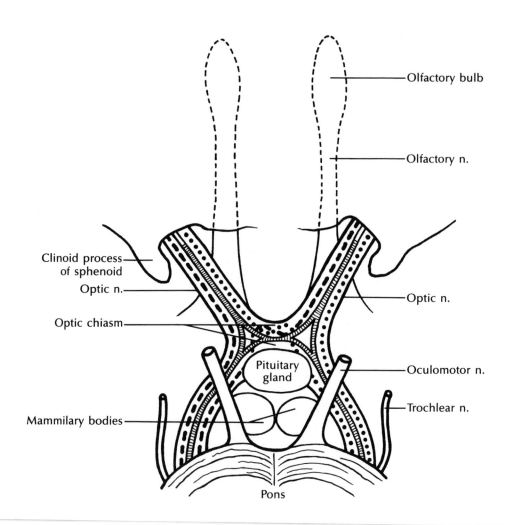

Illustration 1-16
The Optic Chiasm

The hypothalamus is superior and posterior to the optic chiasm. The infundibulum, a downward projection from the floor of the hypothalamus, is directly posterior to the chiasm and gives rise to the pituitary stalk which connects to the pituitary gland. Given these anatomical relationships, it is easy to understand how sphenoidal dysfunction can lead to dysfunctions of vision, endocrine function, appetite and temperature regulation.

The floor of the third ventricle of the brain is also superior to the optic chiasm, and is quite thin. Many small arteries arising from the Circle of Willis converge on the hypothalamus in this area, supplying surrounding brain tissue and following the pituitary stalk downward.

The pituitary gland lies within the sella turcica, a cavity in the body of the sphenoid which is marked by four clinoid processes at its superior corners. The anterior and posterior walls of the sella are bone; the lateral boundaries are formed by the cavernous sinuses. Dural membrane lines the sella and forms the diaphragma sellae through which the pituitary stalk passes (ILLUSTRATION 1-17). The pituitary gland is protected and kept in place by the diaphragm and by fusion with the membrane lining the sella.

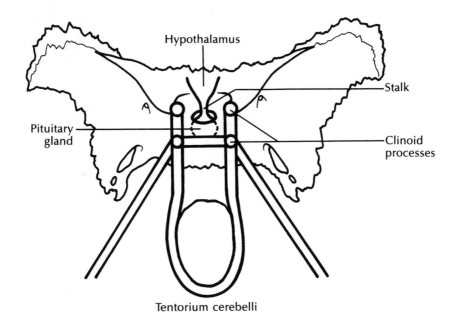

Illustration 1-17
Diaphragma Sellae and Associated Structures

The two posterolateral continuations of the visual sensory axons as they leave the optic chiasm are called the optic tracts. As noted above, each optic tract contains axons from both optic nerves; thus, information from both eyes will still reach the cerebral cortex even if one optic tract is destroyed. Each optic tract projects about 2.5cm straight posterolaterally, then arcs in a more posterior direction as it passes laterally to the cerebral peduncles. Here the optic tract divides into medial (small) and lateral (large) roots, which terminate respectively in the superior colliculus of the midbrain and the lateral geniculate body of the thalamus. The superior colliculus is involved in visual reflexes. The lateral root, though composed primarily of afferent visual sensory axons, also contains a few efferent fibers originating in the brain and terminating in the retina which are apparently involved in responses of the retina to light stimuli.

The afferent fibers of the lateral root (carrying visual sensory information) synapse in the lateral geniculate body with neurons which then send fibers through the occipital portion of the internal capsule of the brain. These fibers form the geniculocalcarine tract which projects to the occipital visual cortex of the cerebrum.

A clinical illustration of how the optic nerve can serve as a pathway into the brain involves a male patient in his 70's whom I treated while I was in general practice. The man demonstrated increasingly bizarre changes in cortical function accompanied by some mild epileptiform seizures. Historically, he received gold shots for treatment of syphilis following World War I. In the 1940's, he received penicillin therapy as a "safeguard." He denied showing any subsequent symptoms of syphilis.

In the 1960's he came under my care for several years for treatment of coronary insufficiency, emphysema, functional gastrointestinal problems and an anxiety-depression complex. He developed CNS symptoms which at first seemed to be transient ischemic attacks. Cerebrovascular dilators, oxygen therapy and anticoagulatives had no effect. He continued to show a positive VDRL, but this was not surprising in view of his history.

His condition continued to worsen, while defying diagnosis by EEG, brain scan, carotid angiograms and neurological consultation (CT scan was not yet available), and he died after two years of progressive deterioration.

Autopsy revealed that *Treponema pallidum,* the causative agent of syphilis, had lain dormant in the vitreous humor of his eye for 30 to 40 years. As the environment became more favorable for some reason, the bacteria became active again, traveled via the optic nerves to the brain and created an abscess which ultimately killed him. This case taught me never to underestimate the longevity of bacterial and viral organisms; I never suspected the true problem before the autopsy.

B. Central connections of the optic tracts

These central connections (ILLUSTRATION 1-18) include the pretectal fibers which travel to the accessory (or Edinger-Westphal) nucleus, which is actually the superior medial part of the oculomotor nucleus and as such supplies efferent stimulation to the oculomotor nerve (III) and the ciliary ganglion, one of the parasympathetic ganglia to be discussed in section III.E.1.

The efferent parasympathetic fibers from the accessory nucleus are responsible for pupillary constriction in response to bright light striking the retina. They synapse at the ciliary ganglion which is located inside the orbit. The oculomotor nucleus is also part of a visual reflex loop which allows us to track and focus on a moving object. The sensory part of this loop is provided by optic nerve input to the oculomotor nucleus, the motor part by fibers to the rectus muscles.

As noted in section III.A.4, the medial root of the optic nerve supplies afferent fibers to the superior colliculus, a gray and white laminated structure located in the corpora quadrigemina of the dorsal midbrain. These afferent fibers synapse within the superior colliculus and send projections to the reticular formation, substantia nigra,

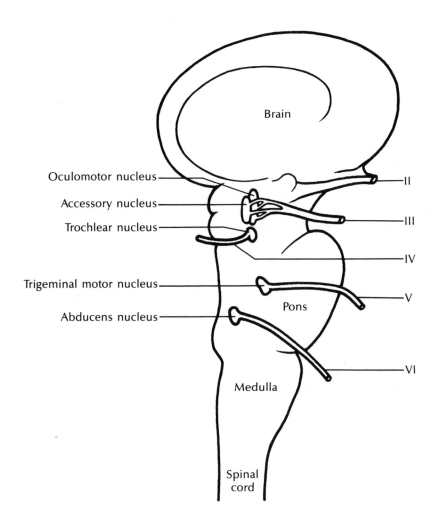

Illustration 1-18
Accessory Nucleus in Relation to Nuclei of
Cranial Nerves II-VI

pons, zona incerta and the tectospinal and tectobulbar tracts which connect to other spinal and cranial tracts. These connections provide the basis for most visual reflexes; e.g., the reticular formation is involved in reflex alertness to visual images which demand attention, and the pons in postural reflexes.

There are projections from the lateral root of the optic nerve, via the lateral geniculate body of the thalamus, to the occipital visual cortex of the cerebrum, as mentioned in section III.A.4. There are numerous association tracts between the visual cortex and other parts of the cerebrum. Complex integrative processes and phenomena such as conscious visual awareness, interpretation, reading, decision-making and memories evoked by current visual input are localized in the cerebrum.

C. Craniosacral system and the visual sensory system

Certain inherent vulnerabilities of the visual system are evident from the anatomic relationships of the optic nerves, optic chiasm and optic tracts. The intraorbital dural sheath of the optic nerve, if under tension from the sphenoid or tentorium cerebelli, or simply lacking sufficient slackness, can produce visual dysfunction and/or restricted eyeball mobility.

I presently have one patient whose symptoms point toward too much tension on the intraorbital optic nerve and its meningeal sheath. When she attempts to move her eyes in a full range of motion to either side, she experiences pain in the occiput at about the level of the posterior occipital protuberance, spreading laterally 5-10cm in both directions. This seems to be a bizarre syndrome until one considers the possible effect of excess tension upon the meningeal sheaths which surround the intraorbital optic nerve. This tension could be created by extreme eyeball movement. If the sheaths have less than adequate "slack," it seems reasonable that restricting tensions might be broadcast to the sphenoid via the firm attachments of the sheaths at the optic foramina. These tensions might then be transmitted from the sphenoid, via the tentorial attachments at its clinoid processes, to the posterior attachment of the tentorium cerebelli located on the occiput, which is precisely where the pain sensation is localized.

The internal carotid artery emerges (bilaterally) from the cavernous sinuses next to the sella turcica. The ophthalmic artery branches off at the level of the anterior clinoid processes, then passes immediately into the orbit through the optic foramen. In the foramen, the artery is inferior and lateral to the optic nerve. It passes to the medial wall of the orbit, where it runs beneath the superior oblique muscle and divides into the frontal and dorsal nasal arteries. An enlargement of this arterial system at any point can interfere with the visual system (SECTION III.A.3).

Along its course, the ophthalmic artery supplies the superior oblique muscle and gives off ethmoid, lacrimal, zygomatic, medial palpebral and ciliary branches. It also gives rise to the central retinal artery which supplies the optic nerve. This artery arises just inside the optic foramen and pierces the dural sheath of the optic nerve shortly after its origin; thus, excess tension on the sheath can interfere with blood transport within the artery and thereby lead to optic nerve dysfunction and deterioration.

Mention has already been made of possible interference with visual system function by pressure or inflammation of sphenoid and ethmoid sinus air cells (SECTION III.A.3), or pituitary gland enlargement (SECTION III.A.4). It should also be kept in mind that the periosteal lining of the orbit is continuous with the dura mater of the cranial cavity; thus, abnormal tension on the dura within the cranium may affect the orbit, and vice versa.

From these facts, it is an inescapable conclusion that normal dural membrane tensions and sphenoid mobility are essential to good visual system function. Occipital and temporal bone mobility are likewise essential to normal tensions in the tentorial dura mater.

Proper functioning of the entire musculoskeletal system, especially the upper cervical vertebrae and the sacrum where there are bony attachments of the dura, is essential to normal functioning of the visual system. This point is illustrated by a case I handled as an osteopathic student. Like many students, I was moonlighting for a local osteopathic GP, in this case one who was noted for his skill in manipulative technique. An ophthalmologist (also an osteopath) referred an 8-year-old girl to the office for osteopathic manipulative treatment of the upper cervical area. The girl's visual acuity had been measured as 20/200 in both eyes. Unbeknownst to me, the ophthalmologist was in the habit of referring such patients for osteopathic evaluation and treatment of musculoskeletal problems, especially of the neck, before prescribing corrective lenses. I simply evaluated and treated the patient as instructed. I found somatic dysfunction at C2 right (i.e., restricted motion of the second cervical vertebra on the right side). I used a direct thrust technique and was successful in mobilizing the joint. On the next day the girl returned to the ophthalmologist for a recheck of visual acuity. I secretly doubted that my treatment could have any significant effect on such extreme myopia, but later learned to my great surprise that the girl was measured at 20/40, a dramatic improvement.

Since then, I have seen many favorable changes in visual acuity which seem to occur consequent to manipulative correction of cervical motion dysfunction, and even more often following successful correction of craniosacral system dysfunctions. One such case involved a 68-year-old design engineer who decided to come for general craniosacral therapy with no specific complaint. I treated him every two weeks for a period of several months. After a few treatments he told me that his latest glasses had become too strong for him, and that he had switched to his most recent previous prescription. Ultimately, he retraced his steps through three previous prescriptions and found himself to be most comfortable with the glasses prescribed when he was in his early 50's.

Since the dural membrane within the spinal canal normally has firm osseous attachments only at the foramen magnum, the posterior body of C2 and C3 and to the second sacral segment, it does not seem possible to manipulatively treat either the cranium or the upper cervical spine alone without affecting the other via the dural membrane.

D. Functional evaluation of the sensory system

The physiologic condition and function of the optic nerve can be estimated by evaluating the integrity of the visual fields and visual acuity, and by ophthalmoscopic evaluation of the retina.

1. Visual fields. The visual fields can be examined for gross defects by wiggling your fingers around the periphery of each field while the patient fixes the eye being examined straight ahead (e.g., on the examiner's nose). The other eye should be covered (ILLUSTRATION 1-19). By moving your fingers around and questioning the patient, you can localize "blind spots" in the visual field.

In general, a visual field defect involving only one eye indicates a problem with the optic nerve between the eyeball and the optic chiasm. Tunnel vision (loss of vision in both lateral visual fields) indicates a problem at the optic chiasm, as discussed in section III.A.4 (ILLUSTRATION 1-20).

Problems of the optic tracts or elsewhere between the optic chiasm and visual cortex usually produce homonymous visual field disturbances, i.e., vision loss in the lateral visual field of one eye and medial field of the other eye. The problem will be found on the same side of the head as the eye which displays the medial visual loss (ILLUSTRATION 1-21).

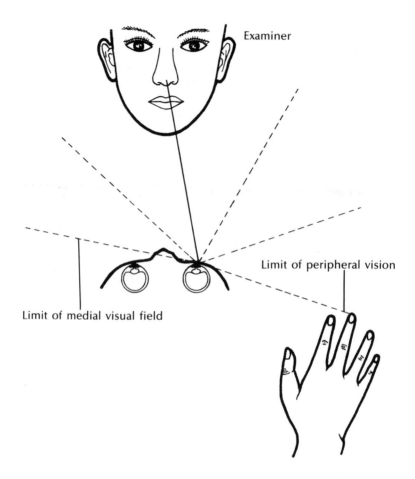

Examiner

Limit of peripheral vision

Limit of medial visual field

Illustration 1-19
Evaluation of Visual Fields

Generally, upper visual field defects suggest problems with the inferior fibers of the optic nerve, and vice versa. This is because light rays cross as they pass into the eyeball through the pupil. Light rays originating from an object in the upper visual field strike receptors on the lower retina. The axons from these receptors generally remain in the lower part of the optic nerve.

Visual acuity is easily examined or screened by use of a standard eye chart. The eyes are examined separately and together at a distance of 20 feet. The line with the smallest print that can be accurately read is noted; numbers (e.g., 20/200, 20/50, etc.) associated with that line provide an index of visual acuity. The "normal" score is 20/20. Various factors (fatigue, somatic dysfunction in the neck, craniosacral dysfunction, toxicity) may interfere with good performance; thus, testing should be repeated on different days and under circumstances designed to minimize the interfering factors.

2. Retina. When you shine the light of the ophthalmoscope through the pupil, you see first what is termed a "red reflex." The anterior chamber is passing light to

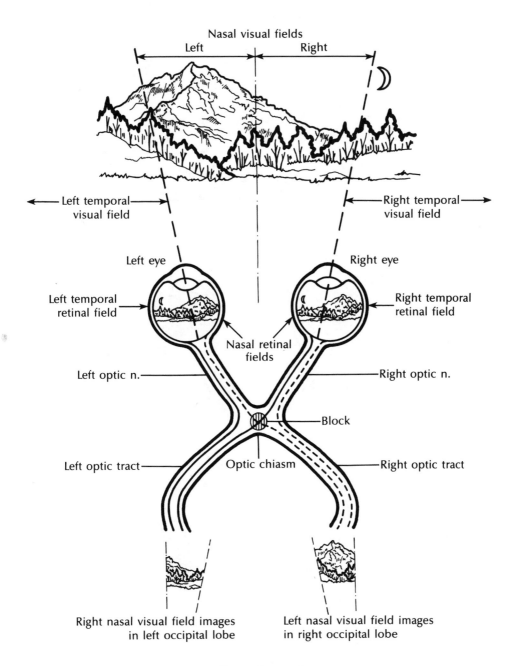

Illustration 1-20
Effect of Lesion at Optic Chiasm

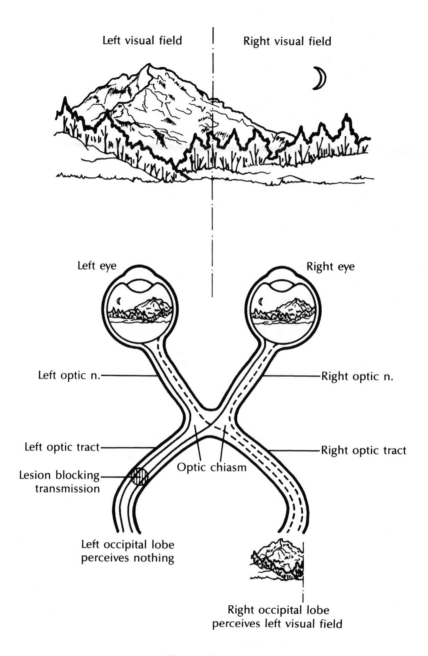

Illustration 1-21
Effect of Lesion of Optic Tract

the retina. This is the same "red reflex" seen in photographs taken with a flash bulb where the subject is looking directly at the camera; the pupils appear red in the photograph.

When using the ophthalmoscope to perform an examination of the retina, you must be sure that there is no interference with the passage of light rays through the anterior parts of the eyeball. It is at this time that cataracts are easily detected. Cataracts are caused by biochemical changes in the normally translucent material of the lens, and are seen as opacities in the body of the lens. As the cataract advances pathologically, it becomes larger and more obstructive. Vision is lost because light rays do not reach the retina. Nothing is wrong with the optic nerve; the photoreceptors are simply receiving no stimulus.

As you look through the pupil, you will be able to see and evaluate the optic disk, retinal arteries, nerves, lens, vitreous and aqueous humors and other structures of the eye. This is a rare opportunity to "look inside" the human body without surgery.

Comparing one eye with the other during this examination is helpful. Study of a photographic atlas of retinae can give you some idea of the appearance of normal and pathologic conditions. But there is no substitute for personal examination of many patients, ideally under the guidance of an experienced ophthalmologist or optometrist. Abnormalities which you are likely to encounter include destruction of veins, redness of the optic nerve, blurring of the disk, exudates and atrophy of the nerve.

When patients complain of severe visual disturbance, hysterical vision loss and malingering must be kept in mind as possible diagnoses. My usual treatment for suspected hysterical loss of vision or paralysis is hypnosis. The hysteria can be suggested away during the hypnotic trance, which will confirm the diagnosis. I do *not* advise the reinstatement of vision or other affected body functions by post-hypnotic suggestion; this simply causes the patient to find other means of expressing the problem. Instead, once the diagnosis of hysteria has been made, you can proceed with an appropriate therapeutic approach.

I am reminded of a puzzling case (it occurred in the late 1960's) of "sudden onset blindness" occurring in a young man shortly before his 18th birthday. The patient was brought to the hospital emergency room by his parents. He stated that he had experienced total vision loss upon awakening that morning but denied any pain or discomfort. I could find nothing pathological upon thorough examination. The pupillary reflex was active; funduscopic exam appeared normal. The corneal reflex was present when touched with the corner of a tissue, but the patient did not blink or flinch when I made a fast move toward his eyes with my hand. He also failed to move his foot when I slowly and deliberately advanced and stepped on his toes. An ophthalmologist friend of mine examined the patient the next day, and could detect neither a pathologic condition nor evidence of malingering.

After consulting privately with my friend, I decided to try some "strategy." Adopting a sad and serious demeanor, I informed the patient that he probably had a tumor which was creating pressure on the optic nerves, and that he would have to return for further testing. Then, without a word, I extended my right hand as if to shake hands with him. He reached out and shook my hand. This dramatic moment concluded the most convincing case of malingering I have ever seen. The patient eventually confessed that he had been feigning blindness in an attempt to evade the military draft.

E. Motor nerves to the eyeball

There are three paired cranial nerves responsible for coordinated motor control of the eyeballs. They have close functional and anatomical relationships and will be considered together. Besides their motor function, they all contain proprioceptive sensory fibers from the muscles they innervate. There are six muscles which move each eyeball (ILLUSTRATION 1-22): four rectus muscles (superior, inferior, lateral and medial) and two obliques (superior and inferior).

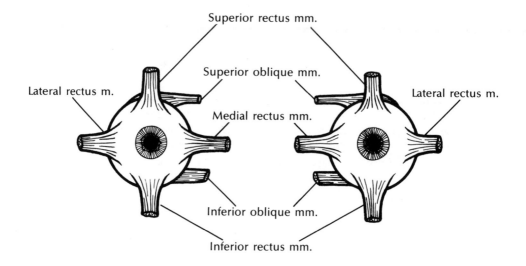

Illustration 1-22
Extrinsic Muscles of the Eye

1. Oculomotor nerve (III). This nerve supplies three of the rectus muscles (superior, inferior, medial) and the inferior oblique. Paralysis of the nerve results in divergent strabismus: the eyeball is aimed laterally. Motion of the pupil is restricted to the lateral and downward directions since only the lateral rectus and superior oblique muscles are unaffected by the condition.

This nerve also contains sensory and motor fibers of the levator palpebrae muscle which raises the eyelid; paralysis of the nerve results in ptosis, or drooping of the eyelid.

The oculomotor nerve conducts parasympathetic axons from the accessory nucleus to the ciliary ganglion (SECTION III.B). This ganglion is located bilaterally between the optic nerve and the lateral rectus muscle in the posterior part of the orbit. It has parasympathetic origin from the oculomotor nucleus, and distributes motor nerves to the ciliary muscle of the lens of the eye and to the muscles of the iris. It therefore has to do with the focusing and pupillary response to light.

The postganglionic fibers of the oculomotor nerve, called the short ciliary nerves, innervate the muscles of the ciliary body and the circular muscles of the iris. Thus, dysfunction of the oculomotor nerve central to its communication with the ciliary ganglion will impair accommodation of the lens and constriction of the pupil.

Finally, the oculomotor nerve receives motor fibers from the sympathetic plexuses of the internal carotid artery and the ophthalmic arteries which branch from it, and conducts these fibers to the eyeball. Most of the sympathetic fibers innervating the eye and related structures originate from thoracic nerves 1-3; they ascend with the cervical sympathetic trunk and synapse in the superior cervical sympathetic ganglion. The functional anatomy of this system is discussed in chapter 2.

2. Trochlear nerve (IV). This nerve supplies only the superior oblique muscle, which moves the pupil downward and laterally. All the fibers of the nerve cross to the opposite side of the body between the central nucleus and the muscle. Thus, dysfunction of one trochlear nerve will affect the contralateral muscle.

3. Abducens nerve (VI). The abducens supplies the lateral rectus muscle, which moves the pupil laterally. Dysfunction of the nerve results in a cross-eyed condition called convergent strabismus. In this case, the nerve fibers do not cross the midline of the body, and dysfunction of one abducens nerve affects only the ipsilateral muscle.

4. Location of nuclei. The nuclei of the oculomotor nerve lie immediately anterior to the nuclei of the trochlear nerve on each side of the midbrain (a short segment of the brain which connects the pons and cerebellum to the forebrain). The nuclei of the abducens are in the pons (located between the medulla and midbrain) just inferior to the trochlear nuclei. Thus, the nuclei for all three pair of nerves are fairly close together (ILLUSTRATION 1-23).

The two oculomotor nerve nuclei are bridged across the midline by a group of cells (called the nucleus of Perlia) which are believed to coordinate convergence of the eyeballs. The oculomotor nuclei are just anterior to the aqueduct of Sylvius which connects the third and fourth ventricles of the brain (ILLUSTRATION 1-24). The nuclei extend forward as far as the third ventricle and send fibers to the tegmentum, red nucleus and substantia nigra. Oculomotor fibers emerge on the anterior brain from the groove between the pons and midbrain, on the medial side of the cerebral peduncles, just posterior to the posterior cerebral arteries, anterior to the superior cerebral arteries and lateral to the basilar artery.

Each oculomotor nucleus is about 8mm long and divided into what one might call "subnuclei." The fibers of these subnuclei project selectively to specific eye muscles. The order of innervation, from anterior to posterior, is levator palpebrae, superior rectus, inferior oblique, medial rectus and inferior rectus.

The trochlear nuclei, as noted above, are just posterior to the oculomotor nuclei. Trochlear fibers travel posteriorly, angling laterally around the central gray matter. They cross in the anterior medulla oblongata and emerge from the dorsal brain surface just below the inferior colliculus of the midbrain. These are the only cranial nerve fibers emerging from the posterior surface of the brain.

These nerves also relate to many arteries as they travel to the eye (ILLUSTRATION 1-25). Problems such as aneurysms or hemorrhages often affect the functions of the nerve which passes near it or which depends upon its blood supply.

The autonomic nuclei are located in a cap-like structure (called the dorsal tegmental nucleus) which covers the oculomotor and trochlear nuclei. This tegmental nucleus includes the accessory nucleus supplying the ciliary ganglia (SECTION III.E.1).

The abducens nuclei are in the pons near the floor of the fourth ventricle, close to the midsagittal plane and just inferior to the trochlear nuclei. The inferior aspect

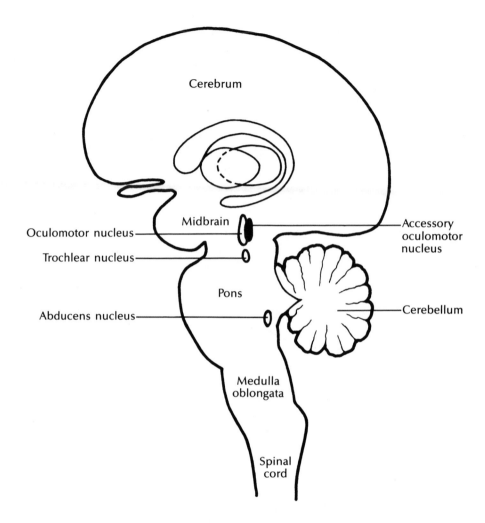

Illustration 1-23
Motor Nerve Nuclei of the Eye

of the abducens nucleus is continuous with the nucleus of the hypoglossal nerve (the motor nerve to the tongue). The significance of this anatomical relationship is open to speculation. My wife once pointed out that one's tongue sometimes tends to move in the same direction as the pupils. This synchrony of movement can be consciously overridden, but the instinctive tendency is definitely there. Perhaps it represents a vestigial behavior from an evolutionary stage in which primates (or their ancestors) used the tongue to taste an object of food, while simultaneously inspecting it visually, before eating.

The fibers from the abducens nuclei travel forward through the entire thickness of the pons between the lateral bundles of the cerebrospinal tracts. They emerge from the furrow between the lower pons and the pyramid of the medulla.

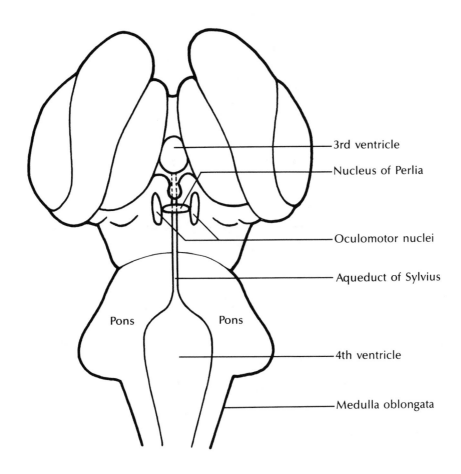

Illustration 1-24
Oculomotor Nuclei and the Nucleus of Perlia

5. Vulnerabilities of the fiber tracts. All three of these nerves exit the brain in the posterior cranial fossa, which is partially divided from the middle cranial fossa by the tentorium cerebelli as it attaches to the petrous ridges of the temporal bones and to the clinoid processes of the sphenoid. The tentorium also provides the superior boundary of the posterior fossa.

The oculomotor and abducens nerves exit from the anterior surface of the brain. The oculomotor fibers do not cross the midsagittal plane. Each oculomotor nerve travels forward in the subarachnoid space within the dural confines of the craniosacral hydraulic system, passing near various arteries (SECTION III.E.4). It crosses the attachment of the tentorium to the posterior clinoid processes, then turns laterally, pierces the dura mater, runs within the dural membrane across the lateral wall of the cavernous venous sinus, and enters the orbit through the superior orbital fissure. As it pierces the dura, this nerve picks up fibers of the sympathetic nervous system derived from the plexus of the internal carotid artery, and communicates with the ophthalmic division of the

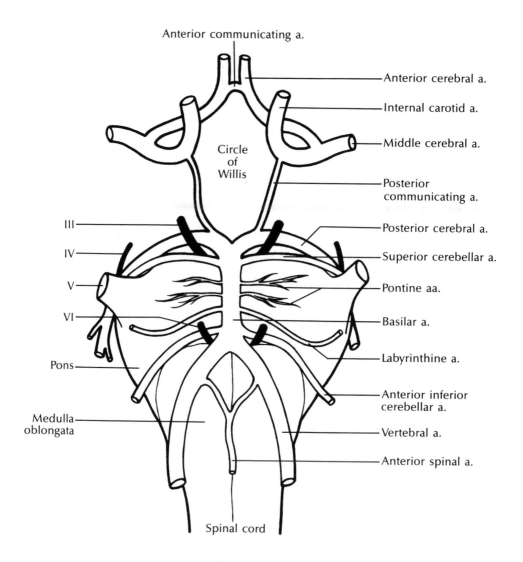

Illustration 1-25
Relationships of Cranial Nerves III, IV and VI
to the Arterial System of the Underside of the Brain

trigeminal nerve (SECTION IV.B). Before passing through the orbital fissure, the oculomotor nerve divides into superior and inferior rami which are invested by dural sleeves upon entering the orbit.

The slender trochlear nerve has the longest course through the subarachnoid space of any cranial nerve due to its posterior exit site (SECTION III.E.4). After its exit from the brain it passes laterally, downward and forward in the transverse fissure between the cerebrum and cerebellum, laterally around the cerebral peduncles and along the underside of the tentorium. The superior cerebellar artery is very close by at this point and can, by enlarging, interfere with function of the nerve. The nerve pierces the dura near the free border behind the posterior clinoid processes and joins the oculomotor nerve. Both nerves then travel along the lateral wall of the cavernous venous sinus and enter the orbit through the superior fissure.

The abducens, shortly after its exit from the medulla, is crossed by the inferior cerebellar artery; enlargement of this vessel can interfere with function of the nerve. The nerve then travels forward and slightly laterally, pierces the dura just lateral to the dorsum sellae (the posterior rectangular part) of the sphenoid body, and runs within the dura over the top of the petrous ridge of the temporal bone behind the base of the posterior clinoid process. It passes over this ridge via a groove in the bone which is converted into a canal by the petrosphenoid ligament; this canal also contains the inferior petrosal venous sinus, usually located medially to the nerve. Also in close approximation to the nerve are the sphenoid air cells, which may exert pressure on it. After crossing the ridge, the abducens joins the trochlear and oculomotor nerves in running through the cavernous sinus and into the orbit (ILLUSTRATIONS 1-26-A and 1-26-B).

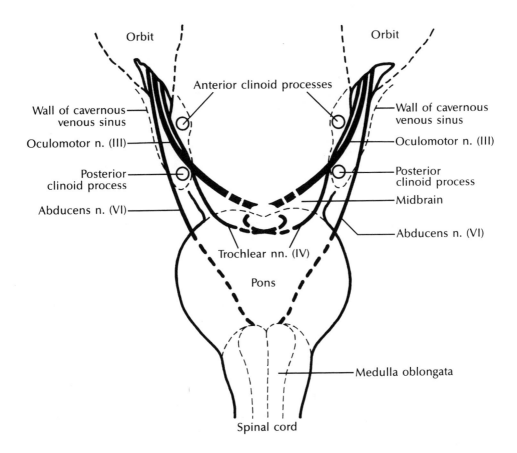

Illustration 1-26-A
Courses of Motor Nerves to the Eye —
Horizontal View

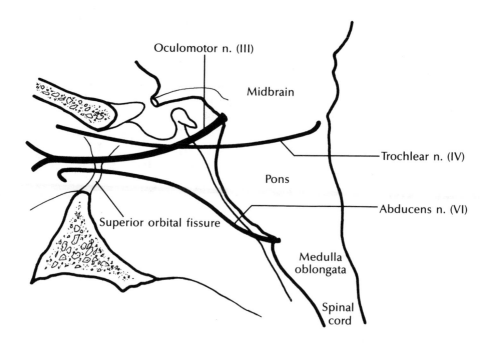

Illustration 1-26-B
Courses of Motor Nerves to the Eye —
Lateral View

F. Cavernous venous sinuses

Since the three nerves discussed in sections III.E and III.G all converge in the cavernous venous sinus after entering the dural membrane, we will digress at this point to consider the anatomy of this paired sinus in some detail.

The cavernous venous sinuses are located bilaterally adjacent to the sphenoid body. They are within the dural membrane and therefore part of the craniosacral hydraulic system. They provide the membranous lateral walls of the sella turcica (SECTION III.A.4). The two cavernous sinuses are connected to each other anteriorly and posteriorly around the stalk of the pituitary gland by two ''intercavernous (or circular) sinuses'' located within the dural membrane tissue which has specialized to form the diaphragma sellae (ILLUSTRATION 1-27).

The cavernous sinuses are part of the larger intracranial venous sinus system which drains most of the blood from the head and provides the reservoir into which cerebrospinal fluid is resorbed by the arachnoid villi. The cavernous sinuses differ from the rest of the system in that they have structural similarities to erectile tissue. For example, they are traversed by many trabeculae which cause movement of venous blood to be slow compared to the other sinuses in the system, and also greatly increase surface area within the cavernous sinuses. This slowing of blood movement and increased surface area tend to increase the likelihood of infection and/or thrombosis. The advantages of the trabecular structure are not clear.

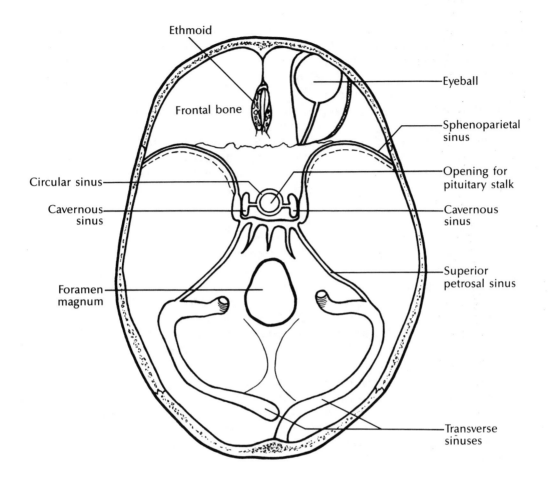

Illustration 1-27
Venous Sinuses of the Cranial Base

The boundaries of the cavernous sinuses are formed by the superior orbital fissure and posterior surface of the orbit (anteriorly); the apex and medial ends of the petrous portion of the temporal bones (posteriorly); the sphenoid, sphenoid sinus air cells and dural membranes lining the sella turcica (medially); dural membrane (laterally and superiorly); and sphenoid (inferiorly).

There are extensive communications between the cavernous sinuses and other venous structures, including: (1) the superior ophthalmic vein (which drains the angular veins of the face) through the superior orbital fissure; (2) the sphenoparietal sinuses (draining the meningeal veins and anterior temporal diploic veins) which run along the underside of the sphenoid lesser wings; (3) the superior petrosal sinuses which exit posteriorly from the cavernous sinuses and run along the petrous ridges of the temporal bones, coming very close to the trigeminal ganglia before they empty into the transverse sinuses; (4) the inferior petrosal sinuses situated in the sulcus formed by the junction of the petrous portions of the temporals and basilar portion of the occipital bone, emptying into the internal jugular veins and venous plexuses located adjacent to the internal carotid artery; (5) the pterygoid venous plexuses through the foramen rotundum, foramen ovale and foramen lacerum; (6) the middle cerebral veins; and (7) the veins which drain the underside of the frontal lobes of the cerebrum.

Because of the interconnections of these venous structures, it is very important that cutaneous infections of the face (boils, pimples, etc.) not be squeezed. Infectious material released in this way can potentially travel via the bloodstream to the cavernous sinuses and cause serious infections there.

The oculomotor and trochlear nerves pass along the lateral walls of the cavernous sinuses, as do the ophthalmic and sometimes the maxillary divisions of the trigeminal nerve. The abducens nerve and internal carotid artery pass more medially within the sinus rather than along its lateral wall. These structures are all separated from venous blood by the dural membrane.

G. Intraorbital course of the three motor nerves

The three nerves discussed in section III.E enter the orbit together through the superior orbital fissure located between the greater and lesser wings of the sphenoid. The fissure is pyramidal in shape, with the apex directed superiorly and laterally; it is bounded medially by the sphenoid body and laterally by the orbital plate of the frontal bone. Other structures passing through the fissure are the trigeminal nerve's ophthalmic division, some sympathetic fibers from the cavernous plexus, the orbital branch of the middle meningeal artery and a recurrent branch from the lacrimal artery running internally toward the dura mater (ILLUSTRATION 1-28).

Each of the three motor nerves picks up a sleeve of dural membrane upon entering the orbit, thereby becoming vulnerable to abnormal dural tensions.

The fissure is located just laterally to the optic foramen (a space between the two roots of the sphenoid lesser wing), through which the optic nerve and ophthalmic artery pass (ILLUSTRATION 1-29).

The oculomotor nerve, as it enters the fissure, passes between the two heads of the lateral rectus muscle which arises from a fibrous ring (annulus tendineus communis) which encircles the posterior orbit and provides an origin for all four rectus muscles. The superior ramus of the oculomotor nerve carries some sympathetic fibers (SECTION III.E.5) and is usually smaller than the inferior ramus. It runs medially, crossing over the optic nerve, and innervates the superior rectus and levator palpebrae muscles. The sympathetic fibers supply smooth muscles of the upper eyelid.

The inferior ramus of the oculomotor nerve splits into three branches. One branch passes under the optic nerve and runs medially to innervate the medial rectus muscle. The second branch runs inferiorly to innervate the inferior rectus muscle. The third branch, running even more inferiorly, supplies the inferior oblique muscle. It also, as it runs between the inferior and lateral rectus muscles, gives off a parasympathetic branch originating from the accessory nucleus and leading to the ciliary ganglion (SECTIONS III.E.1 and 4). This ganglion is 1-2mm in diameter, and located about 1cm from the posterior end of the orbit, just laterally to the optic nerve.

There are two nerve tracts passing through the ciliary ganglion without synapsing: a sensory tract originating from the cornea, iris and ciliary body which eventually joins the ophthalmic nerve in the cavernous sinus, and a sympathetic motor tract originating from the superior cervical sympathetic ganglion and innervating the pupil-

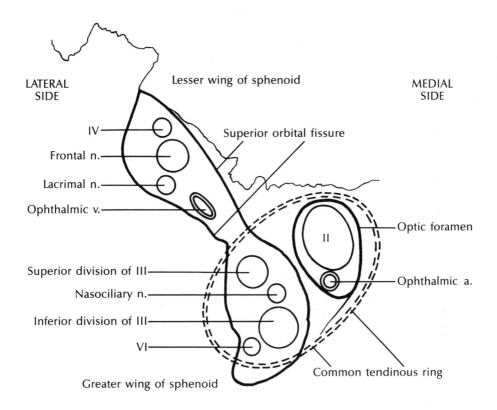

LATERAL
SIDE

Lesser wing of sphenoid

MEDIAL
SIDE

IV

Frontal n.

Lacrimal n.

Ophthalmic v.

Superior orbital fissure

II

Optic foramen

Superior division of III

Nasociliary n.

Inferior division of III

VI

Ophthalmic a.

Greater wing of sphenoid

Common tendinous ring

Illustration 1-28
Posterior View of Left Superior Orbital Fissure
and Its Contents

lary dilator muscles and some blood vessels in the eyeball. The sympathetic fibers which control dilation of the pupil act in coordination with postganglionic parasympathetic fibers emerging from the ciliary ganglion (see preceding paragraph) which accompany the optic nerve and act to constrict the pupil.

The trochlear nerve supplies the superior oblique muscle exclusively. Before entering the orbit, it takes an upward course along the lateral wall of the cavernous sinus, communicates with the sympathetic plexus and ophthalmic nerve and crosses over the oculomotor nerve. It runs above the other nerves as it passes through the orbital fissure. In the orbit, it turns medialward above the origin of the levator palpebrae superioris muscle and penetrates the superior oblique muscle on its orbital surface.

The abducens nerve supplies only the lateral rectus muscle. It passes through the substance of the cavernous sinus rather than running along the lateral wall, and is located laterally to the internal carotid artery and medially to the ophthalmic nerve in this area. It enters the orbital fissure below the other nerves and passes between the two heads of the lateral rectus before penetrating the muscle.

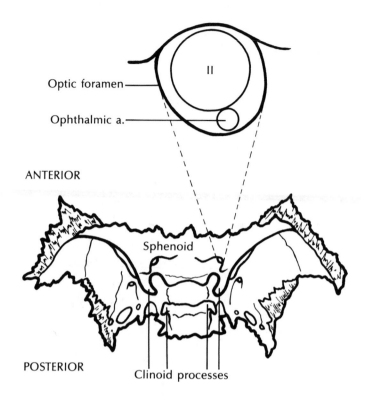

Optic foramen

Ophthalmic a.

ANTERIOR

Sphenoid

POSTERIOR

Clinoid processes

Illustration 1-29
Optic Foramen

H. Craniosacral system connections with the motor nerves

All these motor nerves to the eye carry dural membrane sleeves as they enter the orbit and pass between the superior and inferior layers of the tentorium cerebelli. They are thus all susceptible to abnormal dural or tentorial tension. Recall that both layers of the tentorium are continuous with the falx cerebri at its midsagittal plane, and peripherally with the inner layer of the cranial endosteum (ILLUSTRATION 1-30). The peripheral connection of the inferior layer is with the endosteum of the posterior fossa of the cranial vault, which contains the cerebellum.

The superior layer of the tentorium makes a sling around the anterior clinoid processes of the sphenoid; the inferior layer makes a sling around the posterior clinoid processes (ILLUSTRATION 1-31). Both slings may be considered as extensions of the free border of the tentorium.

All tentorial and falx structures are made of dural membrane. This membrane is tough, waterproof and relatively inelastic. Abnormal tensions from various sources affecting the tentorium at its free borders and at the clinoid processes are certainly capable of interfering with normal function of motor nerves to the eye. Conversely, eye motion dysfunctions can often be corrected by normalizing tentorial tensions. Abnormal tentorial tensions are often traceable to the temporal bones, occiput, upper cervicals and/or sacrococcygeal complex.

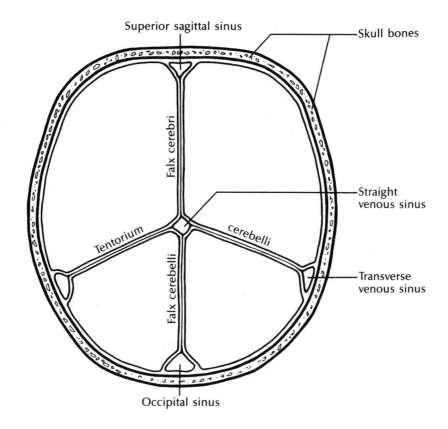

Illustration 1-30
Coronal Section Through Membrane System
of the Cranium

The three motor nerves discussed here are intimately related to the cavernous sinuses. Any problem which increases venous back pressure in these sinuses may contribute to eye motor dysfunction. Since the jugular veins pass through the jugular foramina as they leave the cranial vault, and since these veins carry over 75% of the venous blood from the head into the neck, somatic dysfunction at the foramina can be a significant factor in causing increased back pressure reflected into the cavernous sinuses. The jugular foramina are formed between the occiput and temporal bones 2-3cm lateral to the foramen magnum. Good function of the temporals and occiput is essential to good venous drainage from the head. The tissues at the occipital base must be searched for causes of occipital dysfunction, and the base must be released and allowed to move freely (UPLEDGER 1983: 57). It is also necessary to release the thoracic inlet. Otherwise, the venous back pressure may be increased due to interference with free drainage of blood into the thoracic cage from the veins of the neck (UPLEDGER 1983: 52).

The three nerves pass through the superior orbital fissure, which is formed mainly by the sphenoid; the frontal bone contributes to the lateral boundary. Dysfunction of either of these bones can interfere with function of the nerves and vessels passing through the fissure.

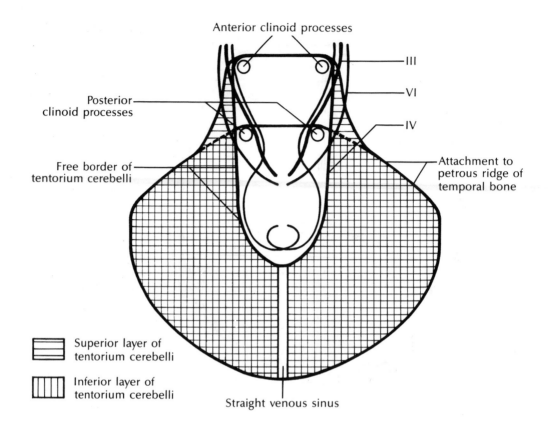

Illustration 1-31
Top View of Tentorium Cerebelli Attachments
to the Clinoid Processes

The ophthalmic vein passes through the fissure along with the three nerves and empties into the cavernous sinuses. Since this vein has no valves, chronic back pressure in the sinuses can result in dilatation of the vein and consequent interference with nerve function.

The three nerves come in contact with numerous arteries, as described in previous sections. Thus, distension, aneurysm, hypertension, abnormal tortuosity and/or abnormal anatomic relationships of the arteries can result in dysfunction of the nerves.

The abducens passes over the petrous ridge of the temporal bone, under the petrosphenoidal ligament. This ligament connects the petrous portion of the temporal to the sphenoid; dysfunction of the bones and tension of the ligament can interfere with abducens function and result in convergent strabismus, probably the most common eye motor dysfunction.

When treating eye motor problems related to craniosacral system dysfunction, you may run into trouble if the patient has had prior eye surgery. If a surgeon has lengthened or partially severed an eye muscle to correct a strabismus and you later correct the craniosacral problem, the eye may then normalize in terms of its motor nerve function, resulting in the opposite type of strabismus.

I had one such experience with a 14-year-old autistic girl. As I corrected her craniosacral problems, she developed a divergent strabismus of the right eye. The medial rectus muscle had been previously operated on for correction of a convergent strabismus in that eye. As the lateral rectus regained its normal strength under my treatment, it overbalanced the weakened medial rectus. The parents decided to continue with the craniosacral therapy because the improvement in autistic behavior was worth the strabismus. In this case the muscles gradually adapted and six months later the strabismus was not apparent. Such adaptation does not always occur, however, and the strabismus may persist. In cases of prior eye surgery, patients and/or their parents should be informed of this possibility before craniosacral therapy is initiated.

I. Structure and function of the eyeball

1. Structure. The ophthalmic nerve, the smallest of the three divisions of the trigeminal nerve (V), is sensory to the eyeball, lacrimal gland, conjunctiva, some of the nasal mucous membrane, skin of the nose, eyelids, forehead, scalp and part of the tentorium. This nerve will be described in greater detail in section IV.B.

The eyeball has many protective devices. The eyebrows offer some protection from sweat dripping down the forehead, and from bright light. The eyelashes guard against the entry of large particles of dust and dirt and help to further diffuse bright light. The eyelids close by reflex when large bodies approach the eye. By blinking, they function in association with lacrimal gland secretions to keep the exposed eyeball surface moist and free of debris (much like the windshield wipers of a car).

The conjunctiva is a transparent membrane which lines the upper and lower eyelids and folds upon itself to cover the surfaces behind the lids. It reduces friction as the lids move over the eyeball, and acts as a barrier against invasion by bacteria.

The lacrimal glands, located under the eyelids, continually secrete a fluid which washes away accumulated dirt, dust and microorganisms from the surface of the eyeball. The eyelid/lacrimal fluid mechanism keeps the eye surface remarkably clean. The fluid also helps prevent infection of eye structures. After washing across the eye surface, the fluid is carried into the nasal cavity by a duct located in the medial corner of the eye opening. Excessive lacrimal fluid secretion (from crying or eye irritation) overburdens the duct and causes the fluid to spill out onto the face, at which point it is called "tears."

Dysfunction of any of the structures mentioned above can potentially result in vision problems. Yet in spite of air pollution, mascara, eye shadow and eyebrow plucking, these protective structures usually function together effectively throughout life.

The tough outer coating of the eyeball is the sclera. It is white, fibrous and provides an insertion site for the six extrinsic eyeball muscles (SECTION III.E.1). It acts as a protective covering for the inner eye structures, and helps maintain the shape of the eyeball. The anterior portion of the sclera, called the cornea, is transparent to allow entry of light waves through the pupil.

Lining the sclera is a membrane called the choroid which carries much of the vascular network of the internal eyeball and is therefore integral in nutrient and metabolite transport. Anteriorly, the choroid becomes the ciliary body which manufactures aqueous humor, a watery fluid filling the anterior chamber of the eyeball (SECTION III.I.2). The aqueous humor is resorbed between the iris and cornea and drains into venous channels. When production exceeds resorption of this fluid, pressure in the anterior chamber rises and glaucoma may result.

Muscles of the ciliary body act on the suspensory ligaments of the lens. One may visualize the lens, ligaments and ciliary body as three concentric circles, the ciliary body being outermost. The lens is flexible and actually consists of about 2,000 layers of tissue, each layer acting to refract light rays passing through to a minute extent. As the concentrically oriented muscles of the ciliary body contract, the outer circle becomes smaller, the suspensory ligaments reduce tension and the lens becomes thicker in its anterior-posterior dimension and smaller in circumference. This change in lens shape allows focusing on nearer objects. When we focus on distant objects, the ciliary body muscles relax, the ligaments exert greater tension and the lens becomes thinner, with a larger circumference. This process of adjusting lens shape is called accommodation.

The choroid is continuous with the iris, a pigmented muscular structure surrounding the pupil and containing both concentrically- and radially-arranged muscle fibers. The iris adjusts the size of the pupil by reflex in response to the brightness or dimness of outside light. Contraction of the concentric muscles reduces pupil diameter, thereby reducing the amount of light entering the eye and striking the retina. The radial muscles of the iris have the opposite effect.

Lining the choroid layer in the posterior part of the eyeball is the retina, containing the photoreceptor rod and cone cells (SECTIONS III.A.1 and 2). The retina and lens form the boundaries of the posterior chamber of the eyeball which is filled with a transparent viscous fluid (vitreous humor) that helps the eyeball maintain its shape and provides a medium for the passage of light rays. Most of the eyeball's mass comes from this fluid (ILLUSTRATION 1-32).

2. Function. When light waves first enter the eye, they are refracted slightly by passage through the cornea; this process is called "coarse focus." The light waves next pass through the aqueous humor in the anterior chamber which is bounded anteriorly by the cornea and posteriorly by the iris and lens. The aqueous humor is normally replaced or "turned over" about every four hours. Occasionally pieces of cellular debris accumulate in the aqueous humor and are perceived as "spots" in the visual field. The light waves then pass through the pupil (which adjusts its diameter in response to external light intensity) and lens (which changes shape depending on focusing distance). Finally, light waves pass through the vitreous humor and strike the photoreceptors of the retina.

As noted in sections III.A.1 and 2, the rods and cones are not distributed homogeneously. The center of the retina, called the fovea centralis, contains only cones and is used for accurate vision in bright light. Cones do not respond well to dim light, making reading and other fine-focus activities difficult. The eyeballs move continuously to ensure that the area of current interest in the visual field always falls on the fovea. The proportion of rods increases as one moves away from the fovea. These photoreceptors are responsive to dim light but do not provide information on color. Thus, our peripheral vision is better in dim light.

Light waves from the external visual field are reversed top to bottom and side to side when they reach the retina. Interpretation of the inverted image takes place in the occipital lobes of the cerebral cortex. Recall that sensory fibers from the medial portion of each retina cross at the optic chiasm, while fibers from the lateral portion

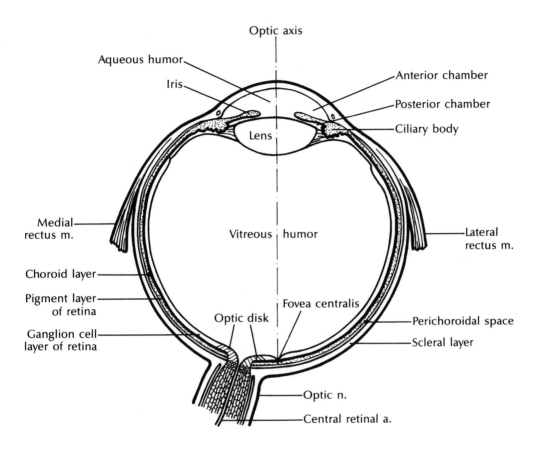

Optic axis

Aqueous humor

Iris

Anterior chamber

Posterior chamber

Ciliary body

Lens

Medial rectus m.

Vitreous humor

Lateral rectus m.

Choroid layer

Pigment layer of retina

Fovea centralis

Ganglion cell layer of retina

Optic disk

Perichoroidal space

Scleral layer

Optic n.

Central retinal a.

Illustration 1-32
The Eyeball — Transverse Section

do not (SECTION III.A.4) (ILLUSTRATION 1-33).

Fibers from the retina join to form the optic nerve (SECTION III.A.2). Within the orbit, the optic nerve is covered by dura mater which blends anteriorly with the sclera. As the nerve passes through the optic foramen in the sphenoid it is fixed and its motion restricted by attachments of the three meningeal layers (SECTION III.A.3).

J. Structure of the orbit

1. Bones. Let us consider the orbit of the eye in greater detail. The bones making up this structure are all accessible to the trained hands of the craniosacral therapist. The orbit is frequently described as pyramidal in shape, with the base consisting of the orbital rim (on the external surface of the face) and the apex represented by the optic foramen. In fact, the shape deviates from a true pyramid in several ways. First, the circumference of the orbit is somewhat larger 1.5cm deep to the rim than it is at the rim itself; this enlargement accommodates the lacrimal gland. Second, the apex of the "pyramid" is displaced somewhat medially, so that it lies roughly on a sagittal

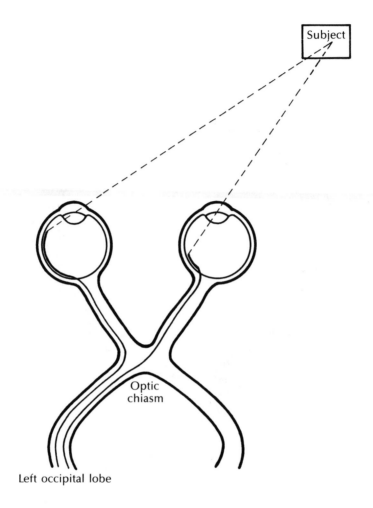

Illustration 1-33
Transmission of Visual Image to Brain

plane directly posterior to the medial wall of the orbit; the medial walls of the two orbits are almost parallel to each other. And third, the medial walls are more quadrangular than triangular in shape (ILLUSTRATION 1-34).

For purposes of the following discussion, we will regard the orbit as consisting of the four inner surfaces illustrated below. This division is somewhat arbitrary and may require use of the imagination.

Bones contributing to the medial wall of the orbit are the frontal (orbital process), lacrimal, ethmoid (orbital lamina) and sphenoid body (which also contributes the medial portion of the optic foramen) (ILLUSTRATION 1-35).

Bones contributing orbital processes to the floor of the orbit are the maxilla, zygomatic and palatine (posteriorly) (ILLUSTRATION 1-36).

Bones contributing to the lateral wall of the orbit are the sphenoid (greater and lesser wings) and zygomatic (frontal process) (ILLUSTRATION 1-37).

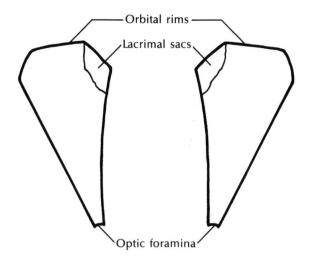

Illustration 1-34
Diagrammatic Top View of Orbits

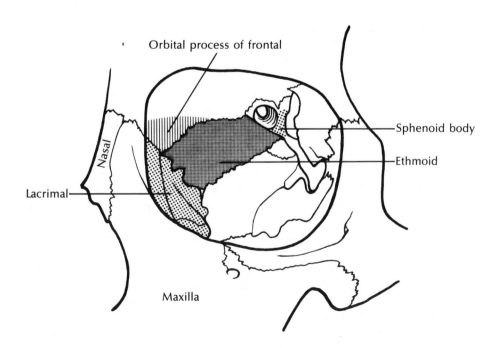

Illustration 1-35
Medial Wall of Orbit

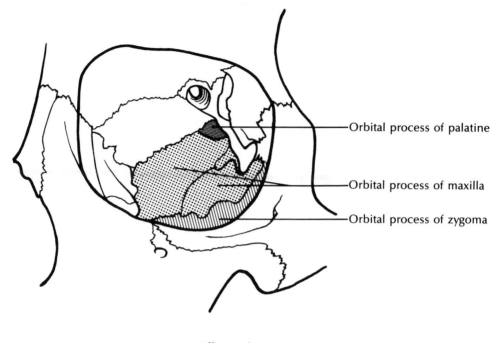

Orbital process of palatine

Orbital process of maxilla

Orbital process of zygoma

Illustration 1-36
Floor of Orbit

The roof consists mostly of the frontal bone's orbital process; the lesser wing of the sphenoid also contributes posteriorly (ILLUSTRATION 1-38).

The ethmoid contribution to the medial wall is extremely thin, and is called the lamina papyracea for this reason. This paper-thin area is the only separation between the ethmoid air cells and the interior of the orbit; an infection of the ethmoid sinus can enter the orbit by this route. Infections can also reach the orbit from the frontal sinuses (which communicate with the ethmoid air cells) or the sphenoid sinuses (since the sphenoid contributes to the optic foramen and posterior portion of the medial wall of the orbit). Considering these relationships, it is clear that the use of craniosacral therapy to mobilize the frontal, sphenoid and ethmoid bones is appropriate to prevent spread of infection through these sinuses and into the orbit. V-spread and vomer techniques are very effective in conjunction with frontal lifts and mobilization of the sphenoid.

The V-spread can be applied from different positions. First, from posterior to anterior. Send from the posterior occipital protuberance through the glabella and, when that has released, angle laterally to treat the frontal sinuses individually. Second, from the inside of the mouth, with the sending finger on the midline and the receiving fingers straddling the glabella. When this has released, move the outside hand laterally to each side in order to treat the frontal sinuses. And third, from the cruciate suture in the mouth by directing the energy up through the coronal suture. This treats the sphenoid sinuses.

In my experience, dysfunction of the ethmoid is best treated by V-spread through it, followed by vomer mobilization and then exaggeration of sphenoid motion. The

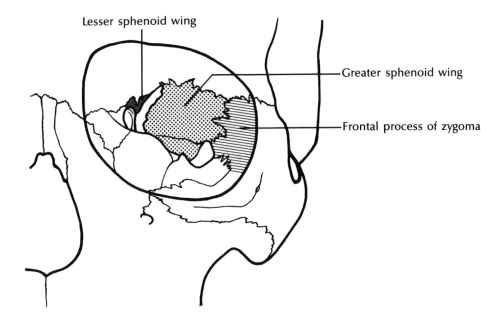

Lesser sphenoid wing

Greater sphenoid wing

Frontal process of zygoma

Illustration 1-37
Lateral Wall of Orbit

frontal lift technique should always be used prior to mobilizing the sphenoid since a restricted frontal can inhibit movement of the sphenoid and render techniques applied to the latter bone less effective.

The floor of the orbit slopes upward medially; there is no real dividing line between it and the medial wall. The lateral boundary of the floor is partially defined by the infraorbital fissure which separates the maxilla from the greater wing of the sphenoid. The infraorbital artery and infraorbital nerves pass through this fissure. The infraorbital artery is a branch of the internal maxillary artery, which in turn branches off the external carotid just below the temporomandibular joint. The infraorbital nerves (derived from the maxillary division of the trigeminal nerve via the sphenopalatine nerves and ganglion) are sensory to the periosteum of the orbital bones. Some filaments pass through the foramina in the fronto-ethmoidal suture and supply the mucous membranes of the ethmoidal and sphenoidal sinuses.

In this context, it is easy to understand the positive effects achievable through mobilization of the maxillae, palatines and sphenoid, and the hard palate techniques described in chapter 12 of my first book. The mobilization of the maxillae and palatines in relation to the sphenoid and its pterygoid processes will affect not only the infraorbital fissure, but also the sphenopalatine ganglion, its nerves and the infraorbital nerves. This will in turn affect the sinuses of the sphenoid, ethmoid and maxillae; some of these sinuses are separated from the orbits by a layer of bone less than 0.5mm thick.

The lateral wall of the orbit is partially delimited from the roof by the superior orbital fissure which is formed between the greater and lesser wings of the sphenoid. A variety of important nerves and vessels pass through this fissure (SECTION III.G). Obvi-

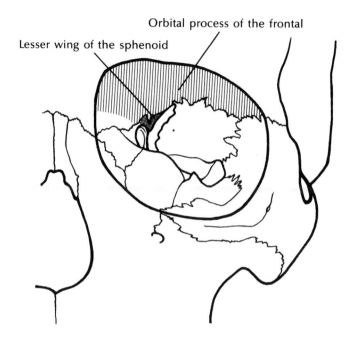

Lesser wing of the sphenoid

Orbital process of the frontal

Illustration 1-38
Roof of Orbit

ously, sphenoid restriction or tension on the dura mater in this region can produce a variety of clinical symptoms. In treating this area, be alert for any sutural restrictions between the sphenoid, frontal and zygomatic bones. I have seen many cases in which restriction of the greater wing of the sphenoid at either the temporal or frontal articulations resulted in rather puzzling orbital/eye pain, frequently coupled with episodic impairment of motor control of the ipsilateral eye when attempting to use the lateral rectus muscle to laterally rotate the eyeball.

The roof of the orbit, consisting mostly of the thin frontal bone, separates the orbit from the anterior cranial fossa. Posteriorly, the lesser wing of the sphenoid separates the orbit from the temporal lobe of the brain. The frontal sinuses cover a large part of the orbital roof; some ethmoidal air cells may also spread laterally into this area.

Thus, the orbit is separated from adjoining sinuses by thin layers of bone on three sides. All techniques which mobilize the orbital bones are appropriate in any case of sinusitis. Stasis encourages the spread of infection (potentially a serious clinical complication) through the sinuses into the orbit.

I treated a 50-year-old male patient whose case history clearly illustrates the possible spread of infection from frontal sinus to orbit. The patient injured his right eye during his teen years; the eye was subsequently removed. He had worn a prosthesis in the right orbit for over 30 years. At the time of consultation, he was suffering an orbital infection with local inflammation and suppuration. He stated that this episode had begun with a "cold" followed by yellow-green discharge from the nose, and moderate pain in the right frontal area of the forehead which progressed to severe pain behind the glabella. The infection then apparently spread to the right orbit and for three days prior to his office visit he had been unable to use his prosthesis. An ophthalmologist had prescribed an antibiotic for more than a week before my exam; this had obviously not succeeded in controlling the spread of the infection.

My examination revealed abnormal restriction of craniosacral motion of the right frontal bone, fronto-nasal and intranasal sutures, vomer, right maxilla and right palatine bone. The right zygomatic area was painful when palpated and there was marked upper cervical somatic dysfunction and tissue contracture which was more prominent on the right side. The thoracic inlet was very tight and required a great deal of effort to achieve a satisfactory release.

It seemed apparent that the spread of infection was via the frontal sinus, through the ethmoid air cells and into the empty right orbit. Treatment consisted of mobilizing all the above structures and releasing the restrictions within 24 hours. The direction of energy technique was also applied through the glabellar region, frontal sinuses and orbit. The sending hand was always placed at the posterior base of the skull.

The infection subsequently cleared within 24 hours. One might question whether this was the result of the antibiotics, rather than the craniosacral treatment. In fact, both therapies probably contributed to the patient's recovery.

2. Orbital fascia. The periosteum of the orbit is loosely attached to the bones except at the sutures, foramina and other orifices. It is continuous with the dura mater of the cranial cavity and with the external skull periosteum, which is tightly attached at the orbital rim.

At the lacrimal crest, the intraorbital periosteum splits to form an envelope (called the lacrimal fascia) which contains the lacrimal sac. This fascia forms the periosteal lining of the nasolacrimal canal through which tears pass from the eye to the nasal cavity.

Posteriorly, the orbital periosteum thickens and forms a ring around the optic foramen and the medial part of the superior fissure called the common tendinous ring. This ring provides attachment for the four rectus muscles and is continuous with their fasciae (ILLUSTRATION 1-39). At the optic foramen there is a fusion of these muscle tendons, the periosteum and the dura mater sheathing the optic nerve.

The space between all of the structures within the orbit is filled with adipose tissue, except the space posterior to the rectus muscle fascia which forms a cone in the posterior orbit. This cone acts as a barrier to the transmission of hemorrhagic blood or pus from one compartment to the other within the orbit. The fascia of the eyeball (Tenon's fascia) intervenes between the adipose tissue and the eyeball itself. This fascia is firmly attached to the sclera posteriorly at the entrance of the optic nerve, and anteriorly about 2mm behind the periphery of the cornea. Between these two areas of attachment, the fascia is loosely attached to the sclera by numerous fine trabeculae. The fascia moves with the eyeball; the extrinsic eye muscles attach to it as well as to the eyeball. An artificial eye implanted in the fascial sheath will therefore move in a natural manner under control of the muscles.

The suspensory ligament of Lockwood (attached to the orbit medially and laterally) is a thickened part of Tenon's fascia. It forms a hammock for the eyeball and helps keep it in place. This ligament receives fascial contributions from the sheaths of several of the extrinsic muscles. There are other ligaments derived from the fascia of the

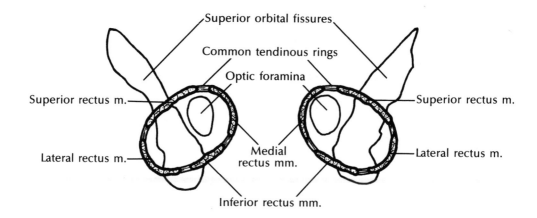

Illustration 1-39
Common Tendinous Ring of the Orbit

extrinsic muscles which tend to maintain the eyeball in its posterior position within the orbit, and to restrict motion.

K. Voluntary muscles of the orbit

There are seven of these muscles, controlling movement of the eyeball and the upper eyelid. The muscles and their innervation were discussed in section III.E. Working together, they allow us to move our eyes about so that we can look at objects which are not directly in front of us, to scan areas of interest and to track moving objects. Movement of the eyeball is generally produced by simultaneous coordinated contraction of some or all of these muscles, never by one muscle working alone.

Since light enters the eyeball through the pupil, and since the fovea centralis (the area of greatest visual acuity) is located directly posterior to the pupil, we get our best visual information when we look directly at the object of interest (SECTION III.I.2). The voluntary muscles help us accomplish this by moving the eyeballs in synchrony without conscious effort.

1. Rectus muscles. The four rectus muscles originate from a fibrous ring (common tendinous ring) which encircles the optic nerve as it enters the orbit through the optic foramen. Laterally, this ring crosses the superior orbital fissure and attaches to a tubercle on the greater wing of the sphenoid. Where they attach to this ring, the tendons of the four rectus muscles blend together. Anteriorly, these muscles attach to Tenon's fascia (SECTION III.J).

Actions of the lateral and medial rectus muscles are straightforward because the origins and insertions are all on the same horizontal plane. For example, as you look to the right, the lateral rectus of the right eye and medial rectus of the left eye act as prime movers, while the medial rectus of the right eye and lateral rectus of the left act in typical antagonist fashion, i.e., exert only enough tension to provide smooth and controlled movement of the eyeballs (ILLUSTRATION 1-40).

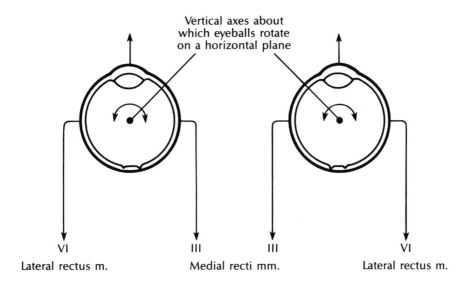

Vertical axes about
which eyeballs rotate
on a horizontal plane

VI
Lateral rectus m.

III
Medial recti mm.

III

VI
Lateral rectus m.

Illustration 1-40
Effect of Medial and Lateral Rectus Muscles
on Eye Movement

The actions of the superior and inferior rectus muscles are somewhat more complicated because the insertions are lateral in relation to the origins; the eyeballs therefore tend to deviate medially in response to contraction of the muscle. To compensate for this tendency, the superior and inferior obliques act in coordination with the superior and inferior rectus muscles, moving the eyeball laterally (SECTION III.K). To understand the actions of the superior and inferior rectus in isolation, visualize an axis of rotation on a horizontal plane through the eyeball such that this axis is perpendicular to an imaginary line from the apex of the orbit through the center of the eyeball. Contraction of the inferior rectus rotates the eyeball downward and medially on this axis. Contraction of the superior rectus rotates the eyeball upward and medially (ILLUSTRATION 1-41).

The levator palpebrae muscle originates from the lesser wing of the sphenoid near the optic foramen; its tendon of origin does not actually attach to the fibrous ring surrounding the foramen but blends with the tendon of the superior rectus muscle. The fibers of the levator muscle run just below those of the superior rectus. These two muscles work together: as the superior rectus rotates the eyeball upward, the levator palpebrae raises the upper eyelid to accommodate this action. The tendon of insertion of the levator muscle broadens into an aponeurosis which attaches to the orbital walls before penetrating the upper eyelid.

Just before this muscle changes to tendon (around the equator of the eyeball) it gives rise on its underside to the superior tarsal muscle, which is sympathetically innervated. Diagnostically this is of interest because if the eyelid droops but maintains the superior palpebral fold, the problem is in the superior tarsal muscle, which is not innervated by the oculomotor nerve. On the other hand, if the eyelid droops and the fold is absent, the problem is either with the levator palpebrae muscle or the superior

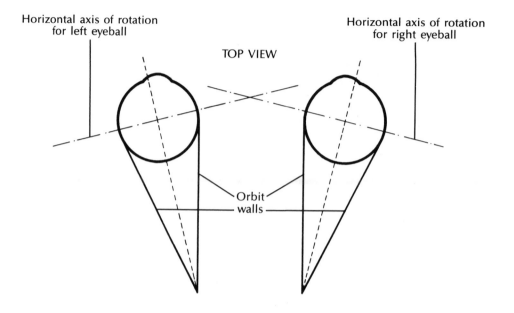

Illustration 1-41
Effect of Superior and Inferior Rectus Muscles
on Eye Movement

branch of the oculomotor nerve. If the eye can aim upward but the lid does not elevate to allow the light to enter the pupil, the problem is in the oculomotor branch to the levator muscle after this branch has left the larger oculomotor trunk, since the innervation to the superior rectus muscle must be intact in order to raise the eyeball. If the oculomotor nerve is dysfunctional before the superior branch is given off, but after the branches to the other voluntary muscles have been given off, the superior rectus and levator muscles will both show paralysis. The eye will not look upward, the eyelid will droop and the fold will be absent.

    2. Oblique muscles. The oblique muscles act to rotate the eyeball around its anterior-posterior axis. This allows the head to be tilted without changing the position of the visual image upon the retina. Both oblique muscles attach to the eyeball laterally: the inferior oblique on the inferior lateral quadrant and the superior oblique on the superior lateral quadrant. Both muscles are oriented in an approximately medial to lateral direction so that contraction results in eyeball rotation around a roughly anterior-posterior axis.

    The superior oblique, innervated by the trochlear nerve, is the longest and most slender of the eye muscles. It originates by a thin tendon above and medial to the optic foramen, just outside the annulus. The muscle changes to tendon before passing through a U-shaped cartilage (the trochlea) which acts as a pulley and allows the tendon to make a sharp turn before inserting on the eyeball. The trochlea is attached by ligaments to spines of the frontal bone. A tendon sheath permits easy movement of the tendon as it passes through the trochlea. The tendon then runs downward, backward and laterally, and inserts on the lateral, superior, posterior quadrant of the eyeball.

Contraction of the muscle rotates the eyeball on its anterior-posterior axis, moving it downward and laterally (ILLUSTRATION 1-42).

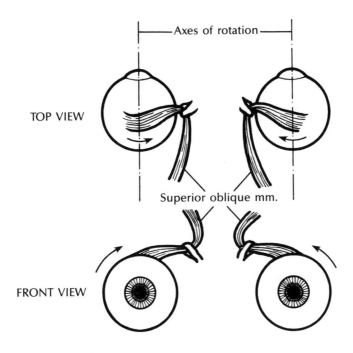

Illustration 1-42
Effect of Superior Oblique Muscles
on Eye Movement

The inferior oblique (innervated by the inferior division of the oculomotor nerve) is the only one of the voluntary muscles of the eye which does not arise from the apex of the orbit. It arises from the orbital surface of the maxilla just lateral to the lacrimal groove. This origin is located in the medial region of the orbital floor, just inside the orbital rim. The muscle runs in a lateral, posterior and upward direction. It passes between the inferior rectus muscle and the orbital floor, then between the lateral rectus muscle and the eyeball. The posterior medial edge of the insertion of the inferior oblique is very near the macula of the retina on the inside of the eyeball. Contraction of the muscle rotates the eyeball on its anterior-posterior axis, moving it upward and laterally (ILLUSTRATION 1-43).

L. Sympathetic innervation to the eye

The sympathetic nervous system acts upon the eye to: (1) dilate the pupil; (2) raise the upper eyelid; (3) vasoconstrict; and (4) inhibit lacrimal secretion. The nerves which enter the eyeball are the nerve of Tiedemann (the plexus around the central artery of the retina), the short ciliary nerves (SECTION III.E.1) and the long ciliary nerves (SECTION IV.B).

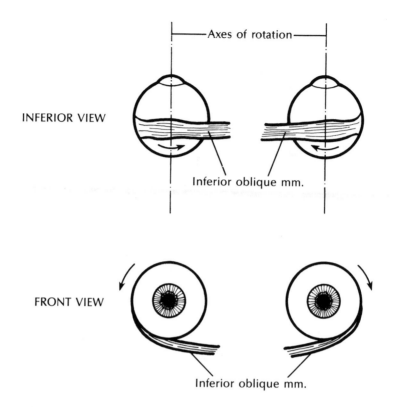

Illustration 1-43
Effect of Inferior Oblique Muscles
on Eye Movement

Paralysis of the sympathetic trunk will produce constriction of the pupil and ptosis (drooping of the eyelid) ipsilaterally. Horner's syndrome (described in 1852 by Claude Bernard and later by Johann Horner) consists of these signs in combination with reduction of intraocular pressure, retraction of the eyeball, absence of sweating (and a secondary rise in temperature) ipsilaterally on the face and neck, hypersecretion of tears, and occasionally facial muscle atrophy and cataract development.

The sympathetic fibers the dysfunction of which are responsible for this syndrome originate in the hypothalamus and do not cross. Some of the fibers, after dividing in the midbrain, pass with the reticular formation through the pons and medulla to the anterior lateral columns of the spinal cord.

After traveling down the anterolateral columns of the upper part of the spinal cord, the preganglionic sympathetic fibers destined to reach the eye exit with the first three thoracic nerve roots. They join the paravertebral sympathetic trunk at their level of exit and then turn upward within the trunk, traveling to the superior cervical sympathetic ganglion. The nerve trunk within which this ascent is made is located on the posterior surface of the carotid artery (within the carotid sheath). The superior cervical sympathetic ganglion (the largest sympathetic ganglion in the body, over 2.5cm long) is located on the anterior surfaces of the transverse processes of C2-4, where it lies between the internal carotid artery and jugular vein. Within the ganglion, the preganglionic fibers which originated from the hypothalamus synapse with postganglionic fibers leading to the eye. As these postganglionic fibers leave the ganglion they join the nerve plexus of the internal carotid artery, traveling with the artery into the skull, through the cavernous venous sinus and (now as part of the ophthalmic artery plexus) through the superior orbital fissure into the orbit. The ganglion provides sympathetic outflow to the internal and external carotid arteries. It is by these arterial plexuses that the sympathetic fibers ascend into the cranial vault with the carotid arteries. The ganglion communicates with the upper four cervical nerve roots and with cranial nerves IX, X and XI. Fibers from the ganglion also enter the pharyngeal plexus, the internal carotid plexus and contribute to the formation of the superior cardiac nerve.

Horner's syndrome may result from lesions in any of these areas, or secondarily from: (1) trauma of the thoracic inlet; (2) pressure on the sympathetic trunk from the first rib due to tumor or abnormal anatomy; (3) upper thoracic surgery; (4) goiter or malignant tumor involving the upper lung or esophagus; or (5) aneurysm with pressure on the sympathetic nerves.

Most of the fibers terminating in the radial muscles of the iris for pupillary dilation leave the arterial plexus before it enters the cavernous sinus. They are diverted to the middle ear with the caroticotympanic plexus, joining the tympanic plexus and possibly participating in auditory/visual reflexes in some way. They then travel with the nerve of the pterygoid canal to rejoin the other fibers in the cavernous sinus, or join the trigeminal ganglion and enter the orbit with the ophthalmic division of the trigeminal nerve.

Once inside the orbit, most of the sympathetic fibers seem to travel with the short ciliary nerves. The fibers to the iris remain with the ophthalmic artery and then join the long ciliary nerves. The fibers leading to the superior tarsal muscle of the upper eyelid may travel with the trochlear nerve. The route of the fibers leading to the lacrimal apparatus is unknown.

The sympathetic fibers to the iris share the long ciliary nerves with sensory fibers from the nasociliary nerve, and with other sympathetic fibers (involved in vasomotor control) from the plexus of the ophthalmic artery.

Sympathetic nerves to the eye are closely integrated with spinal nerve tracts originating from the superior colliculus of the brain and traveling through the brainstem and spinal cord. This integration serves to coordinate spinal reflex activity with pupillary dilation and vasomotor control of ocular blood vessels, facilitating movement of the head and spine as we visually scan the external environment for objects of interest, potential danger, etc.

M. Cleansing system of the eye

The lacrimal, tarsal, ciliary, lymph and trachoma glands all serve to irrigate, cleanse and protect the parts of the eyeball exposed to the outside environment.

The lacrimal glands were introduced in section III.I.1. The superior portion of the gland is located in a fossa in the medial side of the zygomatic process of the frontal bone where it is supported by the tendons of the superior and lateral rectus muscles and a few fibrous bands connecting it to the orbital periosteum. It is about the size and shape of an almond. The inferior (palpebral) portion of the lacrimal gland, which folds around the aponeurosis of the levator palpebrae muscle, is located laterally in the upper eyelid deep to the posterior conjunctiva; it can be seen through the conjunctiva on the everted eyelid.

There are usually between six and twelve ducts from the superior portion emptying into the superior lateral conjunctival fornix. Some of the ducts from the inferior portion empty directly into this fornix; others join ducts from the superior portion. Occasionally, a few lacrimal ducts empty into the inferior conjunctival fornix.

There may be independent accessory lacrimal glands (of Krause) lying deep and adjacent to the conjunctiva. These serve to moisten the cornea even when the major lacrimal glands are not functional. Xerophthalmia (chronically dry cornea) is painful and increases vulnerability to infection of the cornea from dust or bacteria which would normally be washed away.

Because the lacrimal glands lack encapsulation and are intimately related to the frontal bone, malignancy of the glands spreads rapidly to the bone and produces periorbital pain as an early sign.

Blinking of the eyes occurs about every five seconds. Lacrimal fluid accumulates medially on the exposed eyeball, passes through tiny openings in the upper and lower eyelids called puncta, through lacrimal canals and into structures called lacrimal sacs which then drain into the nasal cavity.

The lacrimal sac is 12-15mm long and located bilaterally in the deep groove between the lacrimal bone and the frontal process of the maxilla. It is invested by fascia derived from periosteum at the posterior lacrimal crest of the lacrimal bone and the anterior lacrimal crest of the maxilla.

Abscesses of the lacrimal sac may occur when invading bacteria overcome the antibiotic capacity of the lacrimal fluid. The superior end of the sac (which terminates blindly 3mm above the opening of the lacrimal canal) is covered by the medial palpebral ligament, a barrier seldom penetrated by bacteria. Infection can spread via the nearby angular vein and artery.

A structure called the nasolacrimal duct (15-20mm long) connects the lacrimal sac to the nasal cavity; its entrance into the nasal cavity (located in the inferior nasal meatus) is covered by an imperfect valve formed by a folding of the nasal mucous membrane. The duct lies within a bony canal (which travels downward, backward and slightly laterally) formed by the maxilla, lacrimal bone and inferior nasal concha. The duct is closely fused with the periosteum of these bones.

Nerves and vessels of the lacrimal system are as follows:

- The lacrimal glands receive secretory innervation from parasympathetic fibers derived from the sphenopalatine ganglion; these fibers usually join the lacrimal nerve (SECTION IV.C). The sphenopalatine ganglion (also known as the pterygopalatine ganglion) is a part of the facial system, located in the pterygopalatine fossa just below the maxillary nerve. It supplies parasympathetic secretomotor innervation to the mucous membranes of the nose and palate, as well as the lacrimal glands.

- Sensory innervation to the lacrimal gland is from the lacrimal nerve, the smallest of three branches of the ophthalmic division of the trigeminal nerve. The lacrimal nerve carries its own dural tube and enters the orbit through the narrowest part of the superior orbital fissure (SECTION III.G).

- The lacrimal gland receives its blood supply from the lacrimal artery, which branches off the ophthalmic artery just before its passage through the optic foramen. Branches of the lacrimal artery travel beyond the gland to supply the eyelids and conjunctiva. The anatomic relationships of the ophthalmic artery were discussed in section III.B.
- The venous drainage of the lacrimal glands is into the opthalmic vein.
- Lymphatic drainage is into the conjunctival lymphatics and thence into the parotid lymph nodes which are usually embedded in the parotid glands.
- The nasolacrimal duct system receives blood from the medial palpebral, dorsal nasal, angular, infraorbital and sphenopalatine arteries. The first two are derived from the ophthalmic branch of the internal carotid, the third from the external maxillary branch of the external carotid and the last two from the pterygopalatine branch of the external carotid.
- The veins draining the nasolacrimal system follow the corresponding arteries.
- The nasolacrimal system is innervated mainly by the infratrochlear branch of the ophthalmic nerve (SECTION IV.B), occasionally with contributions from branches of the maxillary division of the trigeminal nerve.

The tarsal glands are modified sebaceous glands located on the inner surfaces of the eyelids and opening onto the free margins of the lids. Their secretion lubricates and protects the conjunctiva, and helps slow down the evaporation of lacrimal fluid on the exposed cornea. There are 25 to 30 of these tiny glands on each eyelid.

The ciliary glands (modified sweat glands) occur in several rows near the eyelashes. They apparently function to keep the lashes and eyelid rims moist.

IV. TRIGEMINAL NERVE

A. Introduction

The trigeminal nerve (V) is the largest in diameter of the twelve paired cranial nerves (the optic nerve is second largest). The trigeminal receives sensory input from most of the face and scalp and from the eyeballs, conjunctiva, lacrimal glands, ear pinnae, external ear canal, nasal cavity, oral cavity, teeth, temporomandibular joint, nasopharynx, meningeal membranes of the anterior and middle cranial fossae and portions of the superior tentorium cerebelli. It receives proprioceptive input from the chewing muscles (temporalis, masseter, pterygoids) and to some extent from the external eyeball muscles and the muscles of facial expression (ILLUSTRATIONS 1-44-A, 1-44-B and 1-44-C).

The trigeminal provides motor innervation to the chewing muscles, mylohyoid, anterior belly of digastric, tensor veli palatini and tensor tympani muscles.

There are three divisions of the trigeminal: ophthalmic, maxillary and mandibular. They provide transportation routes and interconnections for many somatic and autonomic nerves, including other cranial nerves (oculomotor, trochlear, facial, vestibulocochlear, glossopharyngeal, vagus and accessory), four major parasympathetic ganglia (ciliary, sphenopalatine, otic and submaxillary) and the sympathetic plexuses which follow the carotid artery and its branches.

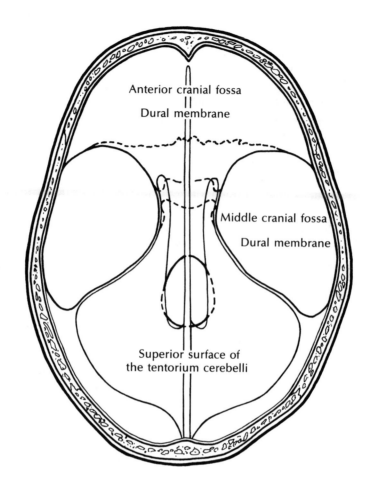

Illustration 1-44-A
Dural Membranes Innervated by the
Trigeminal Nerve

1. Nuclei. The enlarged superior ends of the sensory nuclei of the trigeminal within the brain are called the terminal nuclei. These are located just below the cerebral peduncles which emerge from the lower surfaces of the cerebral hemispheres, and anterior to the cerebral aqueduct which connects the third and fourth ventricles. The terminal trigeminal nuclei pass through the midbrain and enter the pons, at which point they become more slender and are renamed the main trigeminal nuclei. The nuclei continue inferiorly through the pons and medulla, enter the substantia gelatinosa of the spinal cord (at which point they are renamed the trigeminal spinal tract nuclei), continue downward to the level of C2 and then divide into terminals and collaterals (ILLUSTRATION 1-45).

The main trigeminal nuclei receive short ascending branches from sensory areas in the nearby trigeminal ganglia (also called the semilunar or gasserian ganglia). The fibers located in the pons and medulla process pain and temperature sensory input.

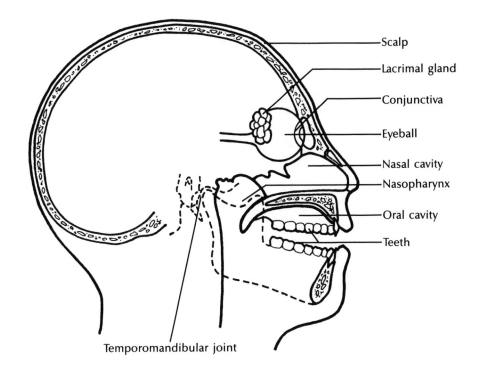

Illustration 1-44-B
Other Areas Innervated by the Trigeminal Nerve

There are numerous interconnections between trigeminal nuclei and other central nervous system tracts. One of these is the reticular activating system (RAS) which helps one react to danger and prepare for appropriate action. This connection may explain the sometimes disproportionate reaction produced by "invasion" of the mouth, nose, etc., by unusual stimuli (e.g., a dentist's drill). There are also connections with motor nuclei in the pons and medulla.

The higher central connections of the trigeminal sensory nuclei are mainly to the post-central gyrus of the cerebral cortex, an important somatic sensory area with close connections to the thalamus. The thalamus is part of the limbic system (SECTION II.C.2) and other central nervous system pathways governing emotional and "primitive" behavior; thus, trigeminal input often plays a part in such behavior. There are also connections to the olivocerebellar tracts connecting the cerebellum to the reticular nuclei (and RAS), and the fasciculus cuneatus (which deals with somesthetic/kinesthetic/ proprioceptive sensory input from the limbs, and localization of skin stimuli). Therefore, these areas are the part of the system which tells us where our left arm is and where the mosquito is biting so that we can smack it accurately without seeing it or thinking about it.

There is a blending of sensory input from the other cranial nerves mentioned above with the ascending trigeminal pathways leading to the thalamus. This integration helps coordinate our responses to stimuli of the face and head.

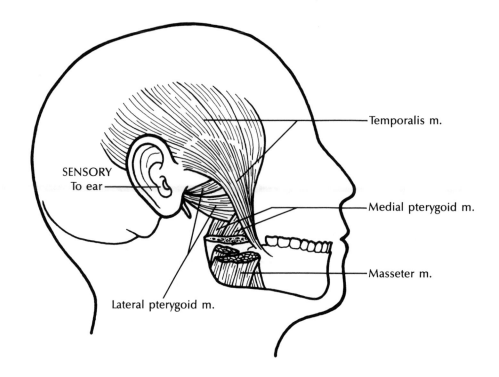

Illustration 1-44-C
Motor Distribution of the Trigeminal Nerve

The trigeminal system includes mesencephalic sensory nuclei on each side of the fourth ventricle. Sensory tracts from these nuclei connect with the motor nuclei of the mandibular division which innervate the chewing muscles; they probably perform a proprioceptive function (to let us know how hard we are biting down).

The cell bodies of the trigeminal sensory nuclei are medium to large in size. Their axons cross to the opposite sides of the brainstem and then form ventral and dorsal tracts. The ventral tracts are well myelinated and run forward through the midbrain to the thalamus after joining the medial lemniscus. The dorsal tracts ascend through the reticular substance (anterior and lateral to the cerebral aqueduct) and then synapse in the thalamus. The post-synaptic fibers run to the "face areas" of the cortex, providing sensory input which influences facial expression in response to pain, cold, etc.

The paired trigeminal motor nuclei are located in the upper pons near the lateral angles of the fourth ventricle, adjacent to the sensory nuclei. They are continuous with nuclei of the facial, glossopharyngeal and vagus nerves. The trigeminal motor nuclei receive input from the trigeminal terminal sensory nuclei (via the trigeminothalamic tracts), corticonuclear tracts, nuclei of the RAS, red nucleus, tectum, medial longitudinal fasciculus, pyramidal tracts and trigeminal mesencephalic roots. All such input is contralateral as well as ipsilateral. It is therefore easy to see why abnormal trigeminal motor responses such as teeth grinding can have so many causes.

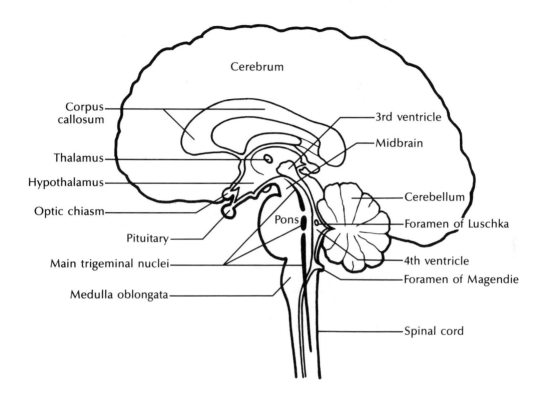

Illustration 1-45
Location of Trigeminal Nuclei

The paired sensory and motor roots of the trigeminal system are located laterally on the middle third of the pons; the sensory root is posterior and inferior to the motor root and is three to five times as large. The sensory root receives input from the various peripheral receptors which transmit this input to the trigeminal ganglion, and from there to the trigeminal nucleus.

The motor root carries a few proprioceptive sensory fibers from the chewing muscles. These sensory fibers are unusual in that they have their cell bodies located within the central nervous system (in the mesencephalic nuclei; see above).

2. Pathways. The distance traveled by the two roots from the pons to the trigeminal ganglion is about 2cm. The two roots travel forward and laterally from the pons, through the subarachnoid space (within the dural envelope) of the posterior cranial fossa and beneath the tentorium. They remain adjacent, but not adhered, to each other; the motor root is generally above and medial to the sensory root. As they cross over the petrous ridge of the temporal bone, they enter a tube-like evagination of meningeal membrane (called the "trigeminal cave") which extends onto the anterior sloping surface of the ridge. On the other side of the ridge is the middle cranial fossa. This cave functions as a sleeve allowing the roots to be bathed in cerebrospinal fluid as they travel from the pons to the ganglion; the design is analogous to the dural sleeves seen around spinal roots. At the trigeminal ganglion the cave fuses to the connective tissue of the ganglion; this fusion provides a barrier ending the peripheral distribution of cerebrospinal fluid. The cave is lateral and posterior to the joint between the temporal apices and the sphenoid, and to the nearby cavernous sinuses (ILLUSTRATION 1-46). It is usually inferior to the superior petrosal venous sinus; in a few cases the cave passes above or through this sinus.

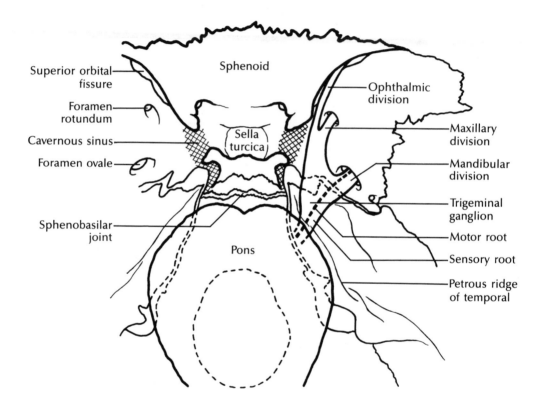

Illustration 1-46
Trigeminal Nerve Between the Pons and Its Exit
From the Cranial Vault

Within each trigeminal cave the ganglion lies on the anterior slope of the petrous temporal. The long axes of this bone run anteriorly and medially and make an angle of about 60° with each other. The mandibular part of the trigeminal ganglion is separated from the carotid artery (running into the middle cranial fossa via the carotid canal) only by a thin layer of dura mater and occasionally bone.

Each trigeminal ganglion is about 1.5cm long and shaped roughly like a half-moon (they are sometimes called the ''semilunar'' ganglia), with the convex side facing laterally. The sensory root leaves from the medial side and the three peripheral sensory divisions of the nerve enter from the lateral side. The motor root does not pass through the ganglion; it passes beneath it and joins the mandibular nerve which leaves the middle cranial fossa via the foramen ovale.

From these anatomical relationships it is obvious that trigeminal ganglion function can be disrupted by carotid artery pressure, venous back pressure or congestion in the cavernous or petrosal sinuses. In such situations, treatment might include mobilization of the temporals, relaxation of the tentorium and opening of venous drainage into the thorax via the thoracic inlet technique and occipital cranial base release technique. The parietal lift with traction, which helps to empty the cranial venous sinus system, may also be helpful.

The great superficial petrosal nerve passes between the trigeminal cave/ganglion complex and the petrous ridge. It has been reported that pressure on this nerve could produce up to 25% reduction in blood flow to the occipital lobe (OWMAN 1977). Such pressure could result from venous back pressure and engorgement of the venous sinuses, or when the tissues around the trigeminal ganglion become swollen or inflamed. Deterioration of visual perception would presumably follow in such a situation. I have frequently seen this phenomenon in my practice. Visual disturbance almost always accompanies acute episodes of tic douloureux, and frequently occurs with impairment of cranial vault fluid outflow at the jugular foramen or thoracic outlet. The techniques mentioned above may improve visual perception in such cases.

In the trigeminal ganglion the fibers of the mandibular division are located laterally, those of the ophthalmic division medially and those of the maxillary division in between (ILLUSTRATION 1-47). As the sensory root approaches the pons it rotates about 120°. As the root enters the pons the mandibular fibers are located superiorly/medially,

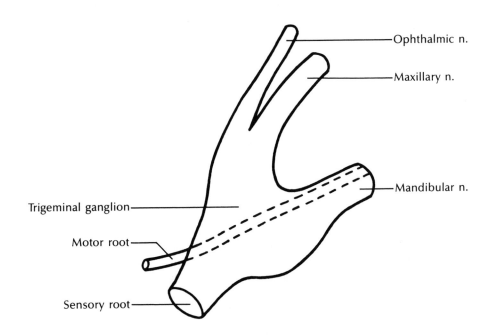

Illustration 1-47
Trigeminal Ganglion

the ophthalmic fibers inferiorly/laterally, and the maxillary fibers remain between the other two.

The three divisions will now be discussed individually, with attention to possible effects of craniosacral therapy techniques.

B. Ophthalmic division

This division of the trigeminal nerve provides sensory innervation to the eyeball, conjunctiva, lacrimal glands, nasal mucosa, paranasal sinuses and the skin of the forehead, eyelids and nose. It exits the trigeminal ganglion from its anterior and medial aspect as the ganglion lies upon the forward slope of the petrous temporal. The flattened nerve trunk then travels 2-3cm within the lateral dural membranous wall of the cavernous venous sinus (where it lies between the oculomotor and trochlear nerves), and enters the orbit through the superior orbital fissure. The nerve is vulnerable to dural strain and venous back pressure as it passes through the sinus.

Within the sinus, the nerve receives sympathetic fibers from the carotid sympathetic plexus, as well as fibers from the oculomotor, trochlear and abducens nerves. Just before passing through the orbital fissure, the ophthalmic nerve sends sensory fibers to the tentorium cerebelli. Within the orbit, the nerve splits into three branches (lacrimal, frontal and nasociliary) (ILLUSTRATION 1-48).

The tentorial fibers leave the ophthalmic nerve and adhere to the trochlear nerve, running posteriorly with it between the layers of the tentorium and providing sensory innervation to the tentorial dura mater. Thus, membranous tension in the tentorium may be felt as pain behind the eyes via the ophthalmic nerve. Treatment in this situation would consist of sphenoido-occipital compression/decompression techniques with traction into the horizontal membrane system.

1. Lacrimal nerve. The lacrimal nerve is the smallest of the three branches of the ophthalmic nerve. It enters the orbit (enclosed in its own dural sleeve) through the narrow superior lateral extreme of the superior orbital fissure, and then runs along the superior border of the lateral rectus muscle and enters the lacrimal gland together with the lacrimal artery. The portion which leaves the lacrimal gland pierces the orbital septum and innervates parts of the skin of the upper eyelid. (The orbital septum is a membranous sheet attached to the edge of the orbit, blending with the tendon of the levator palpebrae muscle and attaching medially to the lacrimal bone.)

Dural tension can interfere with the function of the lacrimal nerve and may be expressed as pain in the upper eyelid, conjunctiva or lacrimal gland. Such restrictions can be located using techniques for evaluation of membrane tension (e.g., asymmetery of cranial motion, arcing or resistance to traction). For dural sleeve restrictions affecting the lacrimal nerve, the V-spread technique must be used in addition to the frontal lift with traction and sphenoid compression/decompression with membrane traction. The V-spread can be applied through the head from occiput to orbit, or from the hard palate to the orbit. It is important that the hard palate be free of restriction itself, since it may drag on the sphenoid via the pterygoid process (most commonly) or through the vomer.

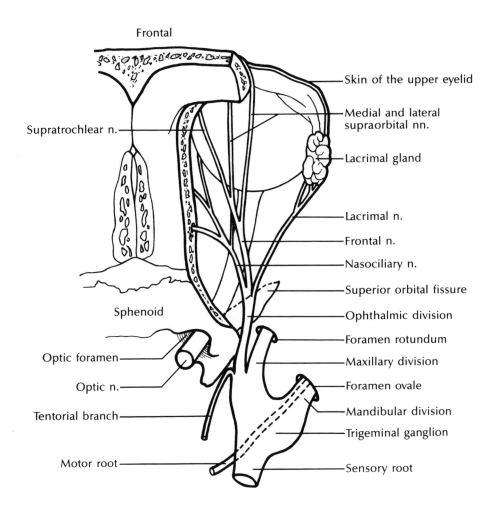

Frontal

Supratrochlear n.

Sphenoid

Optic foramen

Optic n.

Tentorial branch

Motor root

Skin of the upper eyelid

Medial and lateral supraorbital nn.

Lacrimal gland

Lacrimal n.

Frontal n.

Nasociliary n.

Superior orbital fissure

Ophthalmic division

Foramen rotundum

Maxillary division

Foramen ovale

Mandibular division

Trigeminal ganglion

Sensory root

Illustration 1-48
Ophthalmic Division of Trigeminal Nerve

2. Frontal nerve. The frontal nerve is the largest of the three branches of the ophthalmic nerve. Judging from my dissections, it does not carry a dural sheath into the orbit. As it enters the orbit, the frontal nerve is superior to the lateral rectus muscle, superior/medial to the lacrimal nerve, and inferior/lateral to the trochlear nerve. Farther forward, it runs between the orbital roof and the levator palpebrae muscle and splits into two branches, the supratrochlear and supraorbital nerves. The supraorbital is the larger of these two branches. It continues forward through the supraorbital notch (giving off a small branch to the frontal sinus) and innervates the upper eyelid and skin of the forehead. The supratrochlear branch passes medially over the pulley of the superior oblique muscle, communicates with the infratrochlear branch of the nasociliary nerve (see below) and pierces the orbital fascia. It innervates the conjunctiva, the skin of the medial part of the upper eyelid and lower forehead and the corrugator and frontalis muscles.

3. Nasociliary nerve. The nasociliary is the third branch of the ophthalmic nerve. It enters the orbit between the two heads of the lateral rectus muscle, runs forward between the two divisions of the oculomotor nerve, over the optic nerve, under the superior rectus and superior oblique muscles and through the medial wall of the orbit via the anterior ethmoid foramen. As it passes through this foramen, it is renamed the anterior ethmoidal nerve. It enters the cranial vault just above the cribriform plate of the ethmoid, runs along a groove in the plate and passes through the bone into the nasal cavity via a slit-like foramen next to the crista galli. Some fibers innervate the nasal mucous membrane; others emerge between the inferior border of the nasal bone and the lateral nasal cartilage to innervate the skin of the alae and tip of the nose.

As the nasociliary nerve passes between the heads of the lateral rectus muscle, it gives off communicating branches which run laterally to the optic nerve and lead to the ciliary ganglion (SECTION III.E.1). These are sensory fibers from the eyeball which have entered the ciliary ganglion as the short ciliary nerves; they pass through without synapsing, en route to the ophthalmic nerve.

As it travels beside the optic nerve within the orbit, the nasociliary nerve also receives the two or three long ciliary nerves which carry sensory information from the iris and cornea. These nerves pass between the choroid and sclera, penetrate the posterior sclera and pass through the ciliary ganglion without synapse to join the nasociliary nerve.

Sympathetic fibers from the superior cervical sympathetic ganglion (SECTION III.L) "hitch a ride" with the long ciliary nerves, as they have already done with the carotid plexus, the cavernous sinus plexus and the ophthalmic nerve.

Just before the nasociliary nerve passes through the anterior ethmoidal foramen, it gives off a branch called the infratrochlear nerve, which is sensory to the conjunctiva, lacrimal sac, lacrimal carnucle, medial angle of the eye and skin of the eyelids and side of the nose. This nerve runs along the superior border of the medial rectus muscle and communicates with the supratrochlear nerve near the pulley of the superior oblique muscle.

The nasociliary nerve also receives sensory input from the sinuses. A branch called the posterior ethmoidal nerve brings information from the sphenoid and posterior ethmoidal sinuses, and passes through the posterior ethmoidal foramen to join the nasociliary nerve. The anterior ethmoidal branch serves the frontal and anterior ethmoidal sinuses, and joins the nasociliary nerve at the anterior ethmoidal foramen.

The anterior septum, lateral nasal cavity and skin of the alae and nose tip send sensory information via internal and external nasal branches of the nasociliary nerve.

4. Therapy. In terms of craniosacral therapy, the sensory distribution of the ophthalmic division of the trigeminal nerve is of particular interest. It can be used as a means of counter-irritation input into the system. In this way we can encourage the sinuses to drain and actually gain some limited access to the central nuclei. Techniques of counter-irritation include manual pressure, brisk massage, irritant liniments and creams, electrostimulation, needling, etc. V-spread techniques through the pertinent anatomical areas can also be effective. Membrane work is of limited use once the ophthalmic nerve has divided into its three branches and entered the orbit. However, techniques aimed at mobilizing the bones of the orbit (frontal, sphenoid, maxilla, zygomatic, palatines, ethmoid and lacrimal) will be helpful, as will the V-spread technique through the orbit and anterior falx-ethmoid region.

Relations of the rectus and oblique muscles to the trigeminal and other sensory nerves may explain some of the positive effects that eye movement exercises can have upon certain types of headaches, cranio-cervical and facial pain syndromes.

C. Maxillary division

This division of the trigeminal nerve is entirely sensory. It innervates the skin of the middle portion of the face, the lower eyelid, side of the nose, upper lip, mucous membranes of the nose and nasopharynx, maxillary sinuses, tonsils, roof of the mouth, upper gums and upper teeth.

The maxillary nerve leaves the trigeminal ganglion between the other two trigeminal divisions, runs along the anterior slope of the petrous temporal bone, along the lateral wall of the cavernous sinus, through the foramen rotundum and out of the cranial vault. Along this route, it crosses the suture between the sphenoid and petrous temporal, and lies externally to the dura mater. The foramen rotundum is a round tunnel 2.5mm in length in the anterior part of the great wing of the sphenoid.

The normal activity of the maxillary nerve may be compromised by dysfunction of the suture between the petrous temporal and sphenoid, or by excessive dural tension.

1. Pterygopalatine fossa. After passing through the foramen, the nerve enters the pterygopalatine fossa. This is a small triangular fossa (located beneath the apex of the orbit) which also contains the terminal portion of the internal maxillary artery. It is bounded superiorly by the sphenoid body and palatine orbital process, medially by the palatine vertical process, posteriorly by the sphenoid's pterygoid process and anteriorly by the maxilla. Located in the fossa is the sphenopalatine ganglion (SECTION III.M), through which the maxillary nerve passes without synapsing. The maxillary nerve is suspended from the ganglion by communicating branches called pterygopalatine nerves which carry sensory information from the nose, palate, pharynx and posterior teeth (ILLUSTRATION 1-49).

2. Zygomatic branch. A zygomatic branch splits off from the maxillary nerve within the pterygopalatine fossa, and the two nerves run forward together with the infraorbital branch of the internal maxillary artery, passing through the inferior orbital fissure into the orbit, at which point the maxillary nerve is renamed the infraorbital nerve.

3. Superior alveolar branches. The zygomatic and infraorbital nerves travel in a sulcus along the orbital floor, beneath the orbitalis muscle which extends from the inferior fissure to the sulcus. At this point, the infraorbital nerve gives off a middle superior alveolar branch which supplies the middle upper teeth. It then runs forward along the infraorbital canal, gives off another superior alveolar branch which supplies the anterior upper teeth, enters the infraorbital foramen (in the maxilla below the orbital rim) and gives off terminal cutaneous branches. Arterial branches accompany the infraorbital nerve throughout this course. Since the maxillary sinus lies directly below

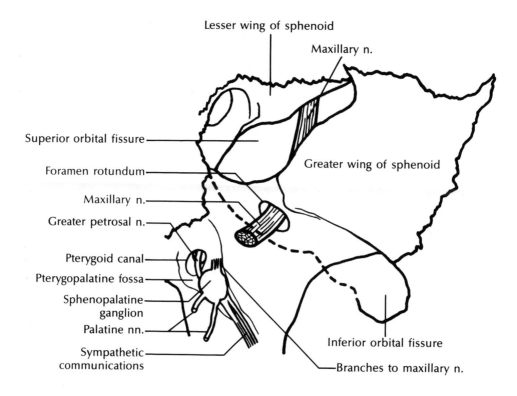

Illustration 1-49
Pterygopalatine Fossa and Ganglion

the orbit, the nerve may be affected by infection or inflammation of the sinus, especially when the bone of the orbital floor is deficient.

The zygomatic nerve diverges laterally from the infraorbital nerve as they run along the sulcus. It splits into two branches on the lateral wall of the orbit; these branches leave the orbit through tiny foramina and supply the skin nearby. In some cases there is also a branch leading to the lacrimal glands; when present, these are parasympathetic secretory/motor fibers "hitching a ride" from the sphenopalatine ganglion.

4. Dysfunction. Normal activity of the maxillary nerve can be affected by dysfunction of the maxilla, palatine, sphenoid, zygomatic or temporal bones, or by abnormal dural tension, tooth-related problems or maxillary sinusitis (which may manifest as eye dysfunction or marked skin hypersensitivity).

D. Mandibular division

This is the largest trigeminal division, and has both sensory and motor function. It arises from the trigeminal ganglion via a large sensory root and a much smaller motor root which travel together downward and through the foramen ovale, at which point the motor root is medial to the sensory root. They immediately join to form the mandibular nerve.

The sensory distribution of this nerve is to the skin or lining of the temporal region, ear, external ear canal, mastoid air cells, cheek, lower lip, lower face, inner cheek, tongue, lower teeth, lower gums, mandible and temporomandibular joint. The nerve supplies motor innervation (plus proprioceptive sensory innervation) to the temporalis, masseter, pterygoid, mylohyoid, anterior digastric, tensor veli palatini and tensor tympani muscles.

The foramen ovale is a hole roughly 1cm in diameter and 2-3mm in length located in the great wing of the sphenoid, posterior to the base of the lateral pterygoid plate and lateral to the foramen lacerum (located in the suture between the sphenoid and petrous temporal). It provides exit from the middle cranial fossa for the accessory meningeal arteries and a branch of the facial nerve (SECTION V), as well as the mandibular nerve (ILLUSTRATION 1-50).

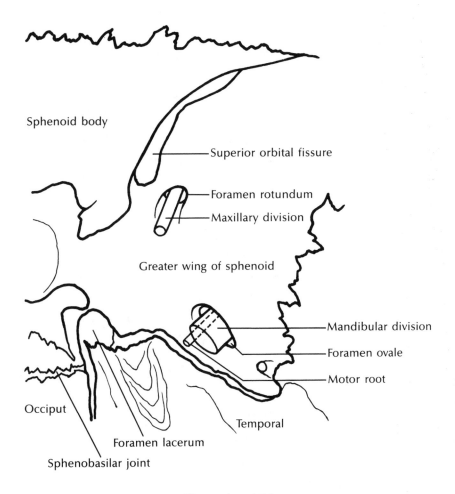

Illustration 1-50
Major Foramina of the Middle Cranial Fossa

The mandibular nerve is just deep to the lateral (external) pterygoid muscle, to which it is intimately related. After 2-3mm, the nerve gives off two branches (nervus spinosus and medial pterygoid nerve), then splits into a posterior and a smaller anterior division. These divisions carry dural sleeves which extend to the skull surface and blend with the periosteum.

In this area, there is close contact between the medial side of the mandibular nerve and the otic ganglion (SECTION V.H). The medial pterygoid nerve frequently passes through this ganglion, but without synapsing.

1. Anterior and posterior divisions. The anterior and posterior divisions of the nerve are separated by the pterygospinous ligament (actually an extension of the cervical fascia) which runs between the lateral pterygoid plate and the spina angularis of the sphenoid (ILLUSTRATION 1-51). This ligament sometimes ossifies.

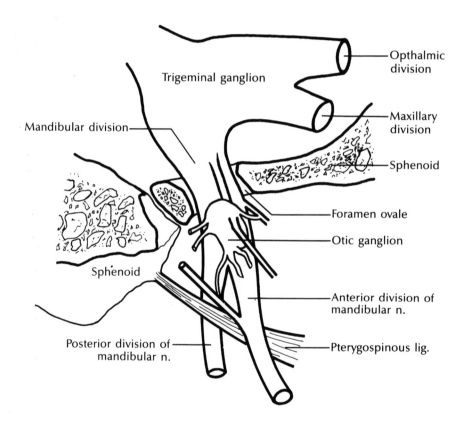

Illustration 1-51
Relations of the Mandibular Division of the
Trigeminal Nerve

The nervus spinosus, along with the middle meningeal artery, reenters the cranial cavity through the foramen spinosum, then splits into two branches which accompany the anterior and posterior branches of the artery and provide sensory innervation to the dura mater and mastoid air cells. The anterior branch of the nervus spinosus communicates with the meningeal branch of the maxillary nerve. The medial pterygoid nerve innervates the muscle of the same name, and sends branches to the tiny tensor veli palatini and tensor tympani muscles (the fibers supplying the latter muscle must pierce the auditory tube).

2. Branches of anterior division. The anterior division of the mandibular nerve has four branches: (1) the masseteric nerve, which is motor to the masseter muscle and sensory to the temporomandibular joint; (2) the deep temporal nerves, usually consisting of two or three subbranches (one may be derived from the buccal nerve); (3) the lateral pterygoid nerve, which diverges from the buccal nerve to supply the lateral pterygoid muscle; and (4) the buccal nerve, which supplies motor innervation to the lateral pterygoid, temporalis and buccinator muscles, and sensory innervation to the skin of the cheek and mucous membrane of the mouth and gums (ILLUSTRATION 1-52). The latter nerve may alternatively arise directly from the trigeminal ganglion (in which case it leaves the cranial cavity through its own foramen), or be replaced by a branch of the maxillary nerve.

3. Branches of posterior division. The posterior division (mainly sensory) of the mandibular nerve has three branches: auriculotemporal, lingual and inferior alveolar (ILLUSTRATION 1-52). The auriculotemporal nerve supplies the external ear, ear canal and tympanic membrane, and communicates with the facial nerve and otic ganglion. It carries postganglionic fibers that synapse with preganglionic fibers within the facial nerve. The lingual nerve communicates with the facial nerve via its chorda tympani branch, and with the hypoglossal nerve via a plexus located anterior to the hyoglossus muscle. The lingual nerve supplies the mucous membrane of the anterior tongue and adjacent mouth and gums. It carries sensory fibers from the taste buds which then pass to the facial nerve, and secretory motor fibers originating in the chorda tympani nerve, synapsing in the submaxillary ganglion and terminating in the sublingual salivary glands. The submaxillary (or submandibular) ganglion is located bilaterally in the tissues of the submandibular salivary glands atop the hyoglossus muscle. It has parasympathetic secretomotor function, and innervates the submandibular and sublingual salivary glands.

The inferior alveolar branch of the posterior mandibular division has four branches of its own. The mylohyoid nerve supplies the mylohyoid and anterior digastric muscles. Dental branches form a plexus in the mandible and supply the molar and premolar teeth. Incisive branches also form a plexus and supply the canine and incisor teeth. Finally, the mental nerve supplies the chin and lower lip, as do portions of the facial nerve.

4. Anatomical relationships significant to the craniosacral therapist. The anatomical relationships of the various branches of the mandibular nerve are important to the craniosacral therapist in terms of diagnosis and treatment. We will therefore discuss them in somewhat greater detail.

The lateral pterygoid muscle, located just outside the mandibular nerve as it leaves the foramen ovale, has a superior and an inferior head, both originating from the sphenoid. The muscle fibers run almost horizontally. The superior head (the smaller of the two) originates from the bottom of the greater wing and from the infratemporal crest

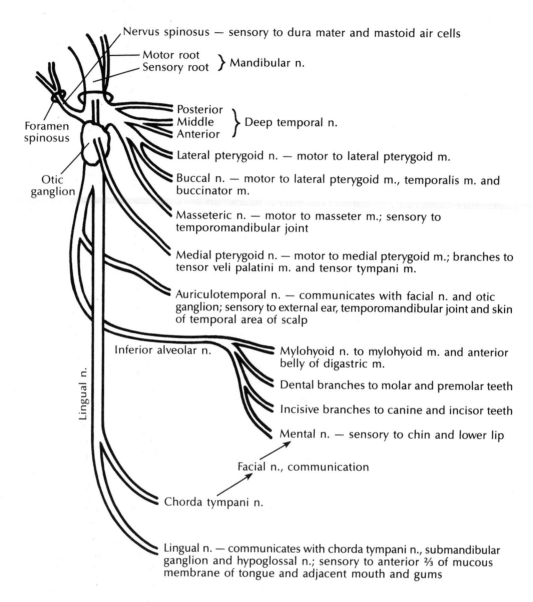

Nervus spinosus — sensory to dura mater and mastoid air cells

Motor root
Sensory root } Mandibular n.

Foramen spinosus

Posterior
Middle } Deep temporal n.
Anterior

Lateral pterygoid n. — motor to lateral pterygoid m.

Otic ganglion

Buccal n. — motor to lateral pterygoid m., temporalis m. and buccinator m.

Masseteric n. — motor to masseter m.; sensory to temporomandibular joint

Medial pterygoid n. — motor to medial pterygoid m.; branches to tensor veli palatini m. and tensor tympani m.

Auriculotemporal n. — communicates with facial n. and otic ganglion; sensory to external ear, temporomandibular joint and skin of temporal area of scalp

Inferior alveolar n.

Lingual n.

Mylohyoid n. to mylohyoid m. and anterior belly of digastric m.

Dental branches to molar and premolar teeth

Incisive branches to canine and incisor teeth

Mental n. — sensory to chin and lower lip

Facial n., communication

Chorda tympani n.

Lingual n. — communicates with chorda tympani n., submandibular ganglion and hypoglossal n.; sensory to anterior ⅔ of mucous membrane of tongue and adjacent mouth and gums

Illustration 1-52
Distribution of the Mandibular Nerve

of the sphenoid and inserts into the articular capsule and disc of the temporomandibular joint. The inferior head arises from the lateral surface of the lateral pterygoid plate and inserts into the pterygoid fovea of the neck of the mandibular condyle and the anterior disc capsule of the temporomandibular joint. Thus, this muscle is roughly triangular, with the three corners of the triangle consisting of the sphenoid, temporomandibular joint and mandible (ILLUSTRATION 1-53).

Chronic hypertonus of the muscle will clearly interfere with sphenoid mobility (i.e., produce a flexion dysfunction). Interestingly, embryologists have stated that a

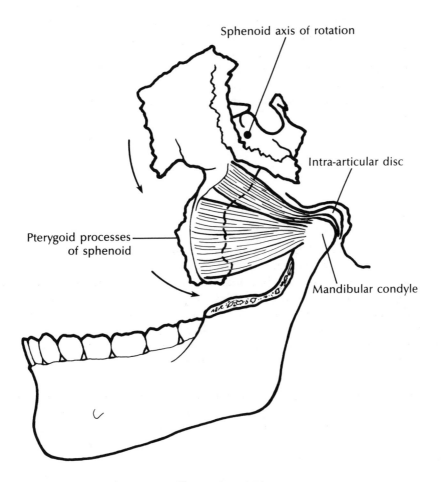

Sphenoid axis of rotation

Intra-articular disc

Pterygoid processes
of sphenoid

Mandibular condyle

Illustration 1-53
Mechanical Effect of Lateral Pterygoid Muscle
Upon the Sphenoid

portion of the tendon from this muscle passes through the temporomandibular joint during development and inserts on the malleus, one of the tiny middle ear ossicles (HARPMAN 1938) (SECTION VI).

The masseteric and deep temporal branches of the mandibular nerve pass above the superior head of the muscle. Sometimes one of the deep temporal nerves passes between the superior and inferior heads. The buccal nerve always emerges between the two heads and travels with the inferior head to the cheek area. The lingual and inferior alveolar nerves run deep to both heads and emerge beneath the inferior head, crossing the external surface of the medial pterygoid muscle.

The maxillary artery passes medially to the mandible and is closely related to some branches of the mandibular nerve. In relation to the lateral pterygoid muscle, this artery may be superficial to both heads, or deep to the inferior head, or may emerge between the two heads en route to the pterygoid fossa.

The trigeminal ganglion and the craniosacral system are so intimately related as to be inseparable. The trigeminal ganglion lies on the anterior surface of the petrous temporal, encased in dural membrane. Its divisions cross the temporal/sphenoid suture and exit the cranial cavity through various openings in the sphenoid bone (inferior orbital fissure, foramen rotundum and foramen ovale). Structures of the trigeminal system, particularly peripheral to the petrous ridge, are vulnerable to excess dural tension and dysfunction of the temporal or sphenoid. Problems with any of these structures can lead to severe clinical symptoms. The craniosacral therapist should therefore pay careful attention to them.

V. FACIAL NERVE

A. Introduction

The facial nerve (VII) has both sensory and motor functions. Its major role is to provide voluntary motor innervation to the muscles of facial expression, the scalp and the external ear, as well as to the buccinator, platysma, stapedius, stylohyoideus and posterior digastric muscles. It also provides: (1) parasympathetic secretomotor innervation to the submaxillary and sublingual salivary glands, lacrimal glands and mucous glands of the nose and palatine areas of the throat; (2) sensory innervation to the anterior tongue (especially for sweet and sour taste perception), external ear canal, soft palate and adjacent pharynx; (3) proprioceptive sensory innervation to all the muscles mentioned above.

Interestingly, there is some anecdotal data suggesting that facial expression (and therefore facial nerve function) in humans can affect one's emotional and psychological state, as well as vice versa. For example, the deliberate assumption of a smiling expression over a period of time might counteract a state of depression. This type of observation raises the question of laughter as a therapy for physical disease or psychological depression. Norman Cousins, former *Saturday Review* editor and medical advisor to the Veterans Administration hospitals, attributed his recovery from a collagen vascular disease and a heart attack to "laughter therapy."

B. Central nuclei

The central origins of the facial nerve are: (1) the facial motor nucleus in the inferior posterior pons; (2) the superior salivatory nucleus (governing parasympathetic secretomotor activity) located just below the motor nucleus; (3) the upper part of the solitary tract nucleus (for sensory taste input from the anterior tongue) located in the upper medulla slightly posterior to the other two nuclei (ILLUSTRATION 1-54).

The motor nucleus receives input from the motor cortex via the pyramidal tracts, as well as from the: (1) corticobulbar tracts; (2) extrapyramidal tracts; (3) tectospinal tracts; (4) reticular formation of the pons (excitatory input); (5) reticular formation of the medulla (inhibitory input); (6) spinal tract of the trigeminal system; (7) solitary tract of the vagus system. With this variety of connections, it is not surprising that the facial nerve system allows us to reflect a wide variety of emotions and sensations through facial expression.

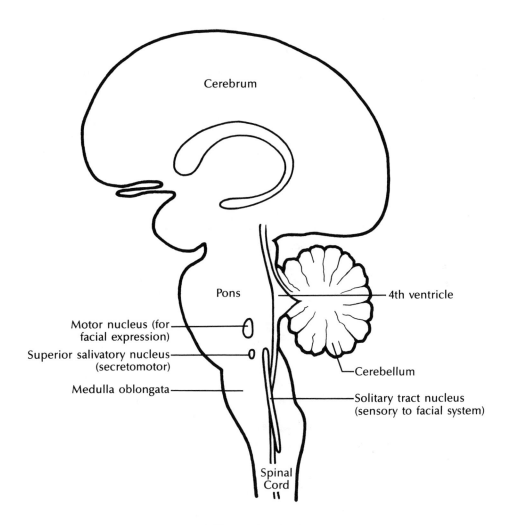

Illustration 1-54
Location of Facial Nuclei

The salivatory nucleus controls secretion of saliva, tears and mucus. It receives input from the vagus system (SECTION VIII) and from the cortex via the dorsal longitudinal tracts.

The solitary tract nucleus which receives sensory taste information from the tongue is actually part of the vagus system; thus, the close interaction between this type of sensory input and the functioning of the digestive system is not surprising.

All sensory nuclei of the facial system are connected to the cortex via the thalamus and medial lemniscus (an ascending fiber tract). There are also, for obvious reasons, reflex connections between the sensory nuclei and the other nuclei (motor and salivary) of the system. The typical facial expressions that accompany emotions such as fear, anger, panic, etc., demonstrate the close connections between the facial system and the reticular activating system.

C. Facial nerve within the subarachnoid space

The facial and vestibulocochlear nerves follow similar courses within the cranial cavity. They exit the brainstem together from the bulbopontine sulcus, a groove located laterally at the junction of the pons, medulla and cerebellum. As they travel away from the brainstem, the large facial motor root remains anterior and superior to the vestibulocochlear nerve root, and the small nervus intermedius (containing the sensory and parasympathetic secretomotor fibers of the facial system) lies in between. These roots run close to the lateral openings of the fourth ventricle (which communicate with the subarachnoid space), to the folds of the choroid plexus (which produces cerebrospinal fluid) and to the anterior inferior cerebellar artery (a branch of the basilar artery).

The three nerve roots travel together laterally through the subarachnoid space, across the base of the occiput near the foramen magnum, across the occipital/petrous temporal suture and into the internal auditory meatus (a total distance of about 2cm) (ILLUSTRATION 1-55-A). At this point the vestibulocochlear nerve diverges from the facial nerve and expands to form the vestibular ganglion (SECTION VI), and the two facial roots join to form a single nerve which continues on into the facial canal.

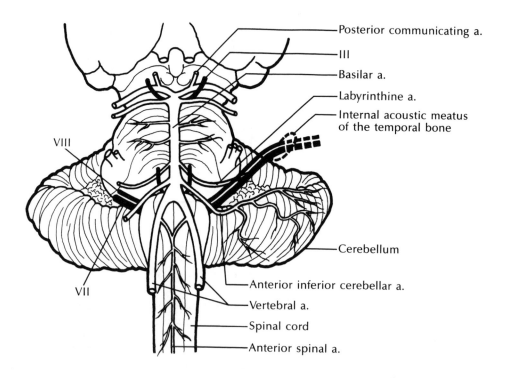

Illustration 1-55-A
Anterior-Inferior View of Cranial Nerves
VII and VIII Between the Brain Stem
and the Internal Auditory Meatus

D. Facial nerve outside the subarachnoid space

The labyrinthine artery (another branch of the basilar artery, supplying the inner ear) accompanies the vestibulocochlear and facial roots into the internal acoustic meatus (ILLUSTRATION 1-55-B).

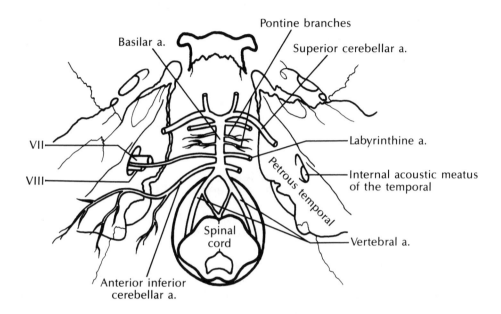

Illustration 1-55-B
Inferior View of Arterial Distribution of the
Brain Stem

The meatus is located on the posterior slope of the petrous temporal about 2cm lateral to the apex and is roughly oval in shape, with a diameter of less than 1cm. It leads to the facial canal. The facial canal continues laterally through the bone for 2cm, turns 90⁰, runs posteriorly/inferiorly for 5cm and terminates at the stylomastoid foramen, located on the inferior surface of the temporal behind the base of the styloid process (ILLUSTRATION 1-56).

At the 90⁰ turn (called the geniculum), the facial canal widens to accommodate the geniculate ganglion, where the sensory fibers synapse. The motor and parasympathetic fibers pass through this ganglion without synapsing. The geniculate ganglion receives taste sensory input from the anterior two-thirds of the tongue. This ganglion is not actually an autonomically functioning nerve structure although many people think of it in that way. It is composed of unipolar cells whose processes bifurcate. The sensory roots pass through the internal acoustic meatus as the nerve of Wrisberg (nervus intermedius) to enter the medulla oblongata. Most of the peripheral branches travel to the taste buds of the anterior tongue via the chorda tympani and lingual nerves (SECTION IV.D). Other branches include sensory to the soft palate which travel via the great superficial petrosal and lesser palatine nerves; sensory to the external ear canal

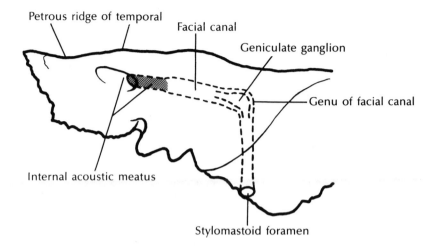

Illustration 1-56
Internal Acoustic Meatus and Facial Canal

and mastoid process which travel via the auricular branch of the vagus nerve; and sensory to the meninges, vasculature and glands.

The parasympathetic fibers pass through the geniculate ganglion and synapse in the more peripheral pterygopalatine and submandibular ganglia. The postsynaptic neurons supply blood vessels, submandibular and sublingual salivary glands, lacrimal glands and some mucous goblet cells of the pharynx and nasal cavity. There are also some facial system fibers exiting the geniculate ganglion which communicate with the otic ganglion via the lesser petrosal nerves, and with the sympathetic plexus of the middle meningeal artery via the external superficial petrosal nerves.

Peripheral to the geniculate ganglion in the facial canal, the facial nerve communicates with the auricular branch of the vagus nerve. Peripheral to the stylomastoid foramen, the facial nerve also communicates with the glossopharyngeal nerve, vagus nerve, great auricular nerve (which ascends from the cervical plexus), auriculotemporal nerve (from the trigeminal nerve mandibular division), lesser occipital nerve and cervical cutaneous nerves.

The facial nerve, after exiting the stylomastoid foramen, runs anteriorly between the temporal styloid process (and the stylohyoid muscle which originates from this process) and the posterior belly of the digastric. It innervates both of the muscles mentioned, and gives off the posterior auricular branch. Less than 2cm after leaving the foramen, the facial nerve crosses over the external carotid artery and retromandibular vein, enters the parotid gland and splits into temporofacial and cervicofacial branches, which then undergo further subdivisions to form a plexus within the gland (ILLUSTRATION 1-57).

E. Vulnerabilities of facial nerve system

The facial system is vulnerable to craniosacral system dysfunction involving the meninges overlying the suture located on the cranial floor between the occipital and

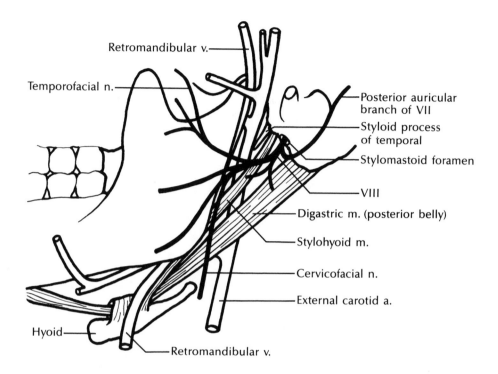

Illustration 1-57
Facial Nerve From Stylomastoid Foramen to
Parotid Gland

petrous temporal bones, or the bones themselves. Such dysfunctions may affect facial expression, salivary function, pharyngeal mucus secretion or cause external ear canal pain. Facial system symptoms may also arise from dysfunction of the temporal bone tissue surrounding the facial canal, the mastoid air cells, the inner and middle ear chambers, or the arteries located near the nerve.

In terms of craniosacral therapy, facial nerve symptoms generally call for diagnosis and mobilization of the occipital and temporal bones and the suture between them. Especially indicated is the temporal "ear pull" technique, followed by mobilization of the temporal on its petrous axis. This is best accomplished by the circumferential treatment technique which rocks the bone on its axis and mobilizes all structures involved, aiding in fluid exchange within the bone and thus preventing stagnation and congestion.

Between the stylohyoid foramen and parotid gland, the facial nerve is vulnerable to compression from the external carotid artery, the retromandibular vein, the posterior digastric muscle, the stylohyoideus muscle, the styloid process of the temporal bone, or the connective tissue structures in the area.

F. Anatomy in the area of the parotid gland

Branching of the facial nerve before it reaches its peripheral target structures occurs within the parotid gland. This gland is located in a fascial pocket formed by splitting of the superficial layer of the deep fascia of the neck. The gland is separated by a thickening of the fascia, called the stylomandibular ligament, which runs from the temporal styloid process downward and forward to the angle and posterior border of the mandibular ramus. This ligament is located between the masseter and medial pterygoid muscles; its deep surface gives origin to some fibers of the styloglossus muscle.

The gland extends over the sternocleidomastoid posteriorly and the masseter anteriorly, behind the mandibular ramus and between the ramus and the temporal mastoid process. It does not pass below the inferior margin of the mandible. It extends up the side of the face, anterior to the ear, to the level of the external ear canal.

Dysfunction of the temporomandibular joint often involves facial nerve symptoms. This joint will be discussed in detail in chapter 3.

G. Other branches of the facial nerve

The great superficial petrosal nerve contains sensory and parasympathetic motor fibers. The sensory fibers supply the soft palate (via the lesser palatine nerves), and to a lesser extent the auditory tube. This branch of the facial nerve emerges at the geniculate ganglion, leaves the facial canal via the fallopean hiatus, emerges in the middle cranial fossa, runs (between the dura mater and bone) in its own groove forward along the anterolateral surface of the petrous temporal, passes under the trigeminal ganglion and exits the cranial fossa via the foramen lacerum, where it runs just lateral to the internal carotid artery. At this point, it unites with the deep petrosal nerve (derived from the carotid plexus) to form the vidian nerve, which then runs forward to the pterygopalatine ganglion. As noted in section IV.A, there is some suggestion of a functional connection between these nerves and blood flow to the occipital cortex.

The pterygopalatine ganglion is a triangular structure, 5mm long, located in a fossa of the same name beneath the maxillary nerve. It is also called the sphenopalatine ganglion (SECTION III.M). The deep petrosal nerve, containing postganglionic fibers from the superior cervical sympathetic ganglion (via the carotid plexus), runs through the pterygopalatine ganglion without synapsing, and supplies the mucous membranes of the nasal cavity and palate via the pterygopalatine branch of the trigeminal system (SECTION IV.C).

In its course between the geniculate ganglion and stylomastoid foramen, the facial nerve gives off a motor branch to the stapedius muscle of the ear, and the chorda tympani (SECTION V.D), which subsequently follows a complex route to the tongue: it doubles back in a separate canal parallel to the facial canal, enters the middle ear cavity through an opening in the lateral wall, passes near the malleus, exits the cavity through a second tiny opening near the anterior border of the eardrum, continues through a canal and emerges from the temporal bone on the medial side of the sphenoidal spine. It then communicates with the otic ganglion and joins the lingual nerve between the lateral and medial pterygoid muscles.

H. Otic ganglion

This is a flattened, star-shaped ganglion, 3-4mm in diameter, lying near the mandibular nerve as it exits the cranial cavity through the foramen ovale. The ganglion is bounded medially by the cartilaginous part of the auditory tube, posteriorly by the middle meningeal artery and anteriorly by the origin of the tensor veli palatini muscle. It is parasympathetic in function, receiving its preganglionic fibers from the inferior salivatory nucleus (located in the medulla) via the facial and glossopharyngeal nerves. The post-ganglionic fibers are secretomotor and supply the parotid gland, mouth and pharynx via the auriculotemporal nerve. The ganglion has non-synaptic connections with the sympathetic plexus of the middle meningeal artery, and with the medial pterygoid and mandibular nerves of the trigeminal system (ILLUSTRATION 1-58).

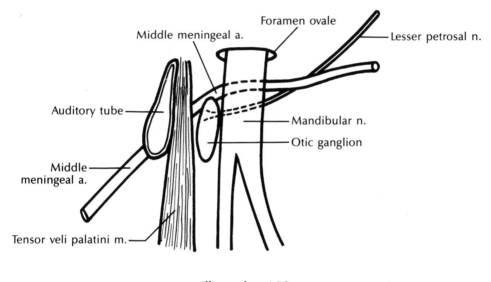

Illustration 1-58
Otic Ganglion

VI. VESTIBULOCOCHLEAR NERVE

A. Introduction

The vestibulocochlear nerve (VIII) consists of two components, the vestibular nerve and the cochlear nerve, with different functions. The auditory function was known before the equilibrial function. The two components also differ in central connections, and in time of myelination during embryonic development. They leave the brainstem separately (the vestibular nerve as a medial root and the cochlear nerve as a lateral root), but always unite as a single trunk before entering the internal acoustic meatus.

Traditional neuroanatomists classify the vestibulocochlear nerve as purely sensory. However, there are suggestions that the two components each contain some motor fibers involved in feedback loops designed to suppress the activity of their respective sensory receptors. These feedback loops could help us adapt to unusual situations (e.g., movement of a ship, weightlessness in space travel, sustained external loud noise) in which continued sensory input to the central nervous system is counter-productive. According to this hypothesis, the motor fibers arise in the superior olive and vestibular nucleus of the central nervous system and pass via the vestibular nerve to the vestibular organs of equilibrium, and via the cochlear nerve to the cochlea (the sensory organ for the sense of hearing).

We will discuss the structure of the vestibulocochlear system by considering each of the two components separately.

B. Components of the vestibulocochlear nerve

1. Vestibular nerve. This component is involved in the sense of equilibrium, maintenance of posture and muscle tone. The cell bodies for the vestibular nerve are bipolar and located in the vestibular ganglion, in the upper lateral portion of the internal acoustic meatus. This ganglion receives sensory input from three branches: superior (supplying the ampullae of the anterior and lateral semicircular canals, and the utricle); inferior (supplying the saccule); and posterior (supplying the ampullae of the posterior semicircular canal, maculae, saccule and utricle). Fibers of these branches leave the vestibule via multiple foramina (ILLUSTRATION 1-59).

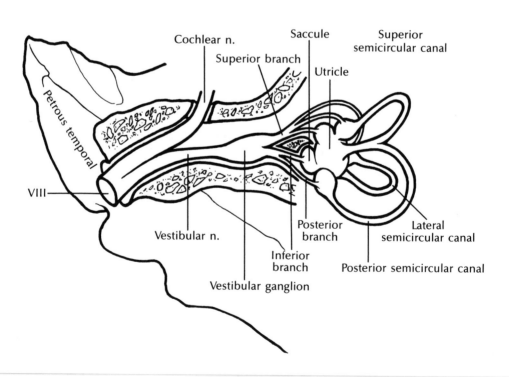

Illustration 1-59
Vestibular Nerve and Ganglion

The sensory receptors for the sense of equilibrium are found in the system of canals and compartments known collectively as the membranous labyrinth, located in the petrous temporal. The labyrinth consists of five interconnected ampullae or vestibules filled with a fluid called endolymph, and containing the receptor cells. Movement of the endolymph through the labyrinth is determined by movement of the temporal bone (and therefore the rest of the skull) in relation to the earth's gravitational field.

There are three semicircular canals, each oriented at 90° to the other two, connected to the utricle. These canals are located posteriorly to the facial canal and medially to the geniculum (SECTION V.D). Each includes an enlarged portion (ampulla) near its junction with the utricle. The ampullae contain structures called cristae which include the sensory cells. The utricle and saccule contain similar structures called maculae. Movement of endolymph within the labyrinth is sensed by hair-like projections from sensory cells in the cristae and maculae, providing the basis for our sense of dynamic (acceleration) and static (positional) equilibrium, respectively.

Once sensory input is received by the vestibular ganglion from the labyrinth, it is relayed to the central nervous system via the central projections of the bipolar ganglion cells. These tracts join with those from the cochlear nerve in the internal acoustic meatus to form the vestibulocochlear nerve.

2. Cochlear nerve. The sensory receptor for the cochlear nerve is the organ of Corti, found in a spiral-shaped structure called the cochlea ("snail"), which is located in the petrous temporal (anterior to the facial canal and medial to the geniculum). It is filled with endolymph. External noise is transmitted in the form of vibrations to the oval window of the cochlea via the external eardrum and the three ossicles of the middle ear.

We may regard the spiral-shaped cochlea as though it were wound around a cone. That cone (about 3mm tall and 6mm in diameter at the base) is called the modiolus. Its apex is pointed anteriorly and slightly laterally. The base would be part of the anterior inferior wall of the internal acoustic meatus. The opening at the apex is called the foramen centrale. Preganglionic sensory fibers from the cochlea pass into the lateral end of the internal acoustic meatus via the foramen centrale or tiny foramina in the lower third of the modiolus (ILLUSTRATION 1-60).

3. Internal acoustic meatus and vestibulocochlear nerve. The internal acoustic meatus is located inside the petrous temporal (SECTION V.D). Within the meatus, the facial and vestibulocochlear nerves run side by side. There are interconnections (the purpose of which is not clear) between the two nerves. A branch (internal auditory) of the basilar artery is also present. A tiny opening (vestibular aqueduct) in the posterior wall of the meatus provides passage for the endolymphatic duct (connected to the vestibular system) and a small artery and vein (ILLUSTRATION 1-61). Pressure on this duct can alter fluid dynamics within the vestibule and affect the sense of equilibrium.

As the vestibulocochlear and facial nerves exit the meatus and enter the subarachnoid space, they are soon joined by the glossopharyngeal nerve. The anterior inferior cerebellar artery is also located in this area; its anatomical relationship to the three nerves is highly variable. The vestibulocochlear nerve runs medially in a fairly straight course to the brainstem. It remains posterior and inferior to the facial nerve. Before reaching the brainstem, it divides once again into its vestibular and cochlear components; the cochlear trunk is usually posterior and inferior to the vestibular trunk. Like

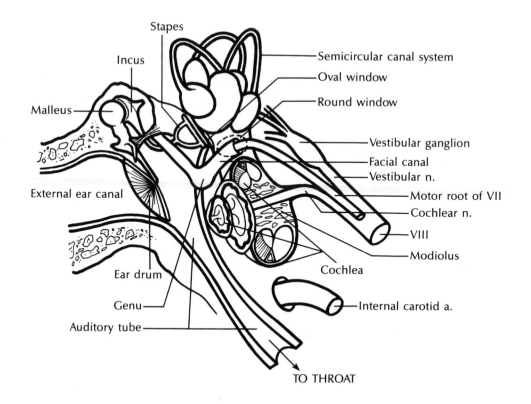

Illustration 1-60
Hearing and Equilibrium Apparatus
in the Petrous Temporal

the two roots of the facial nerve (SECTION V.C), these trunks pass close to the cerebellum and the lateral openings of the fourth ventricle.

C. Central connections of the vestibulocochlear nerve

The cochlear root enters the brainstem lateral to the vestibular root.

1. Vestibular root. This root enters the medulla bilaterally between the inferior cerebellar peduncle and the spinal tract of the trigeminal nerve. It immediately divides into ascending and descending tracts. The descending tract (vestibulospinal root) supplies motor systems which govern the muscles of the neck, trunk and limbs; these systems provide stabilizing reflexes which return the head to its normal position if it is moved. The ascending tract sends fibers to several nuclei in the medulla and lower pons. Some fibers pass directly through the cerebellar peduncles to the flocculomodular nodes of the cerebellum, and are involved in rapid anti-falling reflexes. Other connections between the vestibular nerve and the visual system (SECTION III) help integrate visual/equilibrium information.

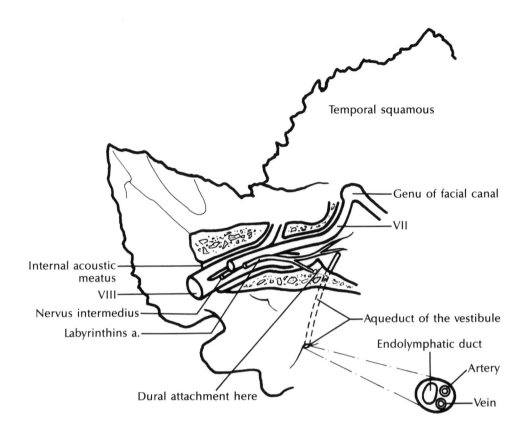

Illustration 1-61
Structures Within Internal Acoustic Meatus

2. Cochlear root. This root is formed by long central processes of the bipolar cells whose bodies are located in the spiral ganglion of the inner ear. The root terminates bilaterally in the ventral and dorsal cochlear nuclei of the medulla, lateral to the inferior cerebellar peduncles and the vestibular nuclei (ILLUSTRATION 1-62). From here postsynaptic fibers cross over and ascend via the lateral lemniscus. There may also be synapses in the inferior colliculus and medial geniculate body; impulses from the latter are relayed to the acoustic areas of the temporal cortex for conscious processing.

There is disagreement about the presence of autonomic innervation within the vestibulocochlear system. My own impression is that both components of the system must contain both sympathetic and parasympathetic pathways.

D. Craniosacral therapy and the vestibulocochlear system

Clearly, craniosacral therapy directed at normalization of temporal bone function is central in problems involving equilibrium and hearing. This does not mean that temporal mobilization will be effective in all such cases, but that it is always worth trying. If nothing else, you will enhance the vitality of the system. I frequently use a V-spread

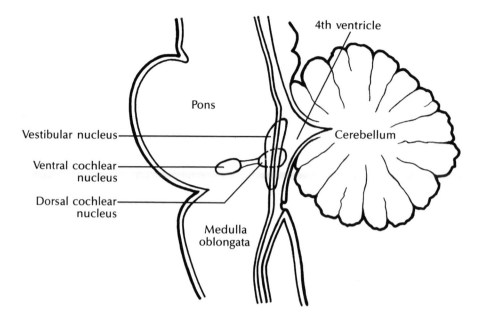

Illustration 1-62
Vestibulocochlear Nuclei

technique through the temporal bones in such patients; the inner and middle ear are not easily accessible by other techniques.

Be sure that the auditory tubes are open and functioning (this involves temporal ear pull techniques, as well as hard palate mobilization), and that the tentorium cerebelli is free of restrictions. In fact, the membrane system should be treated before specific bones are mobilized (except those bones used as "handles" for the membranes).

Simple obstruction of the ear canal can be ruled out in cases of apparent hearing loss by Weber's test. Place the handle of a vibrating tuning fork on the patient's forehead. If the sound is heard best in the "good" ear, cochlear nerve dysfunction is probably present and craniosacral therapy should be employed. If the sound is heard best in the "bad" ear, the external ear canal on that side is probably blocked by wax and the patient should be instructed on cleaning technique.

Similarly, Rinne's test can rule out middle ear congestion. Move the tuning fork away from the ear until the patient can no longer hear the sound, then immediately place the handle against the mastoid process. If the patient hears the sound better through the mastoid than through the air, the hearing loss may be due to middle ear congestion. Hard palate and ear pull techniques may be used in an attempt to open the auditory tube.

VII. GLOSSOPHARYNGEAL NERVE

A. Introduction

The glossopharyngeal nerve (IX) has both motor and sensory functions. It is motor to the stylopharyngeus muscles; secretomotor to the parotid glands and mucous goblet cells on the posterior tongue and pharyngeal wall; and sensory to the pharyngeal mucous membranes, tonsillar beds and fauces, palatine tonsils, taste buds of the posterior tongue, carotid bodies, some blood pressure receptors of the carotid sinus, skin behind the ears, meninges of the posterior cranial fossa, auditory tubes and tympanic cavities.

B. Central nuclei

This nerve arises from several nuclei of the medulla: the nucleus ambiguus and dorsal vagus nucleus (both shared with the vagus nerve), and the inferior salivatory nuclei (part of the reticular formation) (ILLUSTRATION 1-63).

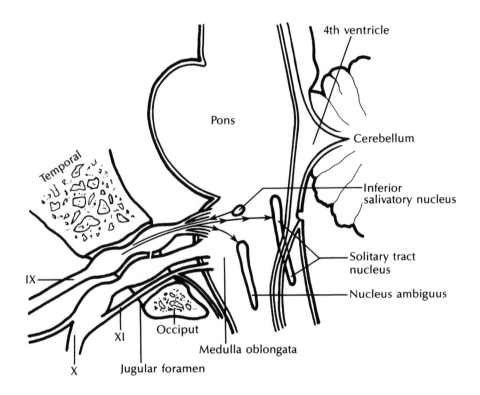

Illustration 1-63
Central Connections of the
Glossopharyngeal Nerve (IX)

Sensory fibers from the posterior tongue terminate in the solitary tract nucleus. Fibers which conduct visceral sensations such as temperature and pain end in the combined dorsal glossopharyngeal-vagal nucleus; those related to general somatic sensation end in the spinal tract and nucleus of the trigeminal nerve.

C. Glossopharyngeal nerve within the cranial cavity

There are three or four rootlets which appear bilaterally at the dorsolateral sulcus of the medulla. These rootlets are in series with the eight or ten rootlets inferior to them, which provide the central connections for the vagus nerve. Immediately after emerging, the glossopharyngeal rootlets converge to form the common trunk known as the glossopharyngeal nerve. The trunk passes laterally across the flocculus to the jugular foramen; en route it is enclosed in its own sheath of dura mater and lies in a groove on the lower posterior portion of the petrous part of the temporal bone. It passes through the foramen laterally and anteriorly to the vagus nerve and the accessory nerve (ILLUSTRATION 1-63).

The posterior inferior cerebellar artery branches off bilaterally from the vertebral arteries before they unite to form the basilar artery. The relationship between the cerebellar artery and the rootlets of the glossopharyngeal, vagus and accessory nerves is variable; it may involve the artery looping around all of the rootlets, part of the rootlets, lying either in front of or behind the rootlets and/or the trunks of the nerves as they are formed by the union of the rootlets. All three of these cranial nerves arise from rootlets which exit the posterior lateral aspects of the medulla bilaterally just below the pons. The rootlets are situated in vertical rows on each side. The upper three or four rootlets form the glossopharyngeal nerve. The vagus nerve arises from the union of as many as ten or twelve of the rootlets. The accessory nerve is usually formed from about five rootlets which unite with the spinal accessory component coming up from the cervical spinal cord through the foramen magnum. The combined nerve exits the cranial cavity through the jugular foramen.

D. Glossopharyngeal nerve within the jugular foramen

The glossopharyngeal nerve remains within the dural sac until it pierces the dural membrane at the jugular foramen. The nerve is the anteriormost structure passing through the jugular foramen. It is separated from the other structures by a connective tissue band which may calcify so that the nerve then actually passes through the foramen in its own bony canal.

Within the foramen, the nerve has two ganglia (superior and inferior). The superior ganglion is quite small (some anatomists think of it as a detached part of the inferior ganglion). Both ganglia are sensory, transmitting sensations of taste (bitter and sour) from the posterior third of the tongue and part of the soft palate; pain, touch and temperature from the posterior tongue, the fauces, the pharyngeal wall and some pain from the meninges of the posterior intracranial fossa; and sensory impulses from the carotid bodies and the carotid sinuses.

There are communications between these ganglia and the vagus nerve, the sympathetic tracts and sometimes the facial nerve (this latter communication occurs more often after the glossopharyngeal has exited from the jugular foramen). Within the foramen, the glossopharyngeal nerve gives off a sensory branch (the tympanic nerve) to the ear.

E. Glossopharyngeal nerve outside the cranial cavity

After exiting the jugular foramen, the glossopharyngeal nerve runs anteriorly between the internal carotid artery and the internal jugular vein, and posteriorly to the styloid process of the temporal bone and all the muscles and ligaments which attach to that process. The nerve runs about an inch along the posterior border of the stylopharyngeus muscle, innervating the muscle as it crosses over it on the superficial side to the hyoglossus muscle (which it does *not* innervate). The nerve then enters the tissues behind the hyoglossus and receives sensory input from the palatine tonsils, posterior pharynx, posterior third of the tongue and the regional glands (ILLUSTRATION 1-64).

1. Tympanic nerve. The tympanic nerve, a branch of the glossopharyngeal nerve, supplies secretomotor parasympathetic innervation to the parotid glands through the otic ganglion, and receives sensory input from the mucous membrane of the middle ear cavity. After separating from the glossopharyngeal nerve, the tympanic nerve has its own tiny canal through the temporal bone between the jugular foramen and the tympanic cavity through which it travels. The tympanic nerve contributes to a tympanic plexus which is formed in conjunction with sympathetic fibers derived from the carotid plexus, and with a branch of the greater petrosal nerve. This plexus receives sensory impulses from the windows of the middle ear cavity, the mucous membranes of the cavity, the ear drum (tympanic membrane), the auditory tubes and the mastoid air cells. Earaches and pain from blocked auditory tubes are mediated almost exclusively via this tiny nerve. The tympanic nerve exits the cavity through a tiny canal and then becomes known as the lesser petrosal nerve.

2. Lesser petrosal nerve. The lesser petrosal nerve, another branch of the glossopharyngeal nerve, reenters the cranial cavity through a canal which ends on the superior ridge of the petrous temporal. This reentry point is just lateral to the opening of the facial canal. The nerve then travels down the anterior slope of the petrous temporal, exits the cranial cavity via the suture between the greater wing of the sphenoid and the petrous temporal, communicates with a nerve from the geniculate ganglion of the facial nerve and terminates in the otic ganglion, to which it supplies parasympathetic input.

3. Otic ganglion. The otic ganglion (SECTION V.H) is variable in contour, and about 3mm in diameter. The medial pterygoid nerve, which arises from the mandibular nerve at its origin, is actually imbedded in this ganglion, but this connection is merely structural, not functional. Recent information suggests that the only functional communication the otic ganglion has (besides the parasympathetic fibers of the lesser petrosal nerve) is with the sympathetic innervation which comes from the carotid and middle meningeal plexuses.

4. Carotid sinus nerve. The carotid sinus nerve branches from the main trunk of the glossopharyngeal nerve just after its emergence from the jugular foramen. The carotid sinus nerve communicates near its origin with the vagus nerve via the inferior vagal ganglion (SECTION VIII.B) (or the vagus-pharyngeal nerve branch). It then travels on the anterior surface of the internal carotid artery to the bifurcation where the carotid sinus is located. Here it receives sensory information about blood pressure which it

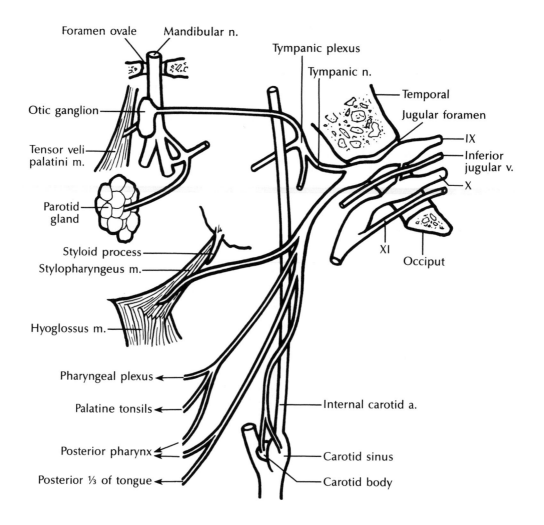

Illustration 1-64
Otic Ganglion and Extracranial Parts
Of Glossopharyngeal Nerve (IX)

transmits back to the medullary nuclei of the trigeminal nerve and the solitary tract, which it shares as a central connection with the vagus nerve. It also receives sensory input from the carotid body, which gives information about oxygen, carbon dioxide and pH levels in the blood.

5. End of the glossopharyngeal nerve. The continuation of the glossopharyngeal nerve combines with the vagus nerve and sympathetics to form the pharyngeal plexus. There are usually three or four paired glossopharyngeal branches to this plexus, leaving the main trunk at the level of vertebra C2.

The only muscle innervated by the glossopharyngeal nerve is the stylopharyngeus. This long, slender muscle originates from the medial side of the base of the temporal styloid process, passes downward between the superior and middle constrictor pharyngeus muscles and inserts on the deep side of the pharyngeal mucosa and the thyroid cartilage (it may blend with the fibers of constrictor muscles). It elevates the pharynx during swallowing, speaking, etc. The terminal branches of the glossopharyngeal nerves go to the tonsils, the tongue, the pharyngeal mucosa and their related glands and taste buds.

F. Craniosacral approach to the glossopharyngeal system

Glossopharyngeal "tic douloureux" is a not uncommon clinical problem. It involves severe pain which is usually episodic and may involve any portion of the sensory distribution of the glossopharyngeal nerve. It may manifest as severe pain in the middle ear, mastoid air cells, tongue and/or posterior pharyngeal wall. The condition is essentially due to hypersensitivity of the glossopharyngeal nerve; the triggers which set off the pain are usually located in the tonsil bed. Treatment is often by surgical intervention: entering the cranial vault via the occiput, the glossopharyngeal rootlets are cut to eliminate sensory pain input. Craniosacral therapy, with focus on release of the jugular foramen, may be successful in these patients although, because you are agitating the glossopharyngeal nerve with your technique, the pain may exacerbate before it gets better. Appropriate techniques may include: (1) release of the occipital cranial base (UPLEDGER 1983: 57); (2) the temporal bone circumferential treatment techniques (UPLEDGER 1983: 179); (3) stabilization of the occiput with one hand while you further mobilize the temporal bone on the involved side (this will further mobilize the occipitomastoid suture, of which the jugular foramen is just a "wide spot in the road"); (4) V-spread technique through the skull at the level of the glossopharyngeal rootlets (this sends energy through from one mastoid process to the other). The tissue is rather dense, so it takes awhile for the therapeutic pulsation to occur in this last technique. Be patient.

Since the glossopharyngeal nerve carries its own sleeve of dura mater into the jugular foramen as it leaves the cranial cavity, any dural restriction involving the endosteum overlying the occipitotemporal region in the cranial floor must be corrected. Such restriction can contribute to glossopharyngeal hypersensitization.

VIII. VAGUS NERVE

A. Introduction

The vagus nerve (X) is another mixed motor/sensory nerve. It is the longest of the twelve cranial nerves, and has the most extensive distribution and functional variability. Its name comes from the Latin word for "wanderer."

The vagus brings sensory information from, and distributes motor fibers to, both visceral and somatic structures. The vagus, in combination with the glossopharyngeal and accessory nerves, makes up a unique system which is mostly parasympathetic in function. These three nerves share the dorsal vagal nucleus, the solitary tract nucleus and the nucleus ambiguus. The vagus also has a functional connection with the trigeminal spinal nucleus.

The somatic sensory portion of the vagus innervates the ear canal and the skin of the posterior external ear. The visceral sensory portion receives input from the pharynx, larynx, bronchi, lungs, heart, esophagus, stomach, large and small intestines and bile duct system. The somatic motor division supplies the larynx, pharynx and palate. Most of this voluntary innervation is shared with the accessory nerve; which of the two nerves supplies a specific structure in a given individual is variable.

The vagus exits the posterior/lateral medulla bilaterally by eight to twelve rootlets, in series with the rootlets of the glossopharyngeal nerve above and the accessory nerve below (SECTION VII.B). All of these rootlets exit between the olive (above) and inferior peduncle (below). The vagus rootlets unite shortly to form the vagus nerve.

B. Central nuclei

The central nuclei of the vagus system are all located in the medulla. The medulla is located directly above the foramen magnum; it connects the spinal cord (below) to the pons of the cerebral diencephalon (above), and to the cerebellum (posteriorly). There is no sharp line of demarcation between the lower medulla and the upper spinal cord. If one arbitrarily selects a boundary at the level of the foramen magnum, the medulla is about 3cm long, 2cm wide and 1cm thick from front to back. It is amazing that this structure transmits almost all of the messages between the brain and the body. About half way up through the medulla, the central canal of the spinal cord enlarges into the fourth ventricle of the brain.

The dorsal vagal nucleus is a longitudinally oriented column of cells with sensory and motor functions, located bilaterally in the floor of the fourth ventricle. It is lateral to the hypoglossal nucleus, and extends the entire length of the medulla. Visceral sensory information is conducted into the dorsal vagal nucleus from the inferior vagal ganglion via the axons of sensory cells which receive information from the respiratory tree and lungs, digestive tract, liver, pancreas, kidneys, heart and aorta. The motor tracts which originate in the dorsal vagal nucleus supply all of those organs which receive sensory supply from these nuclei.

The inferior vagal ganglion (also known as the nodose or petrous ganglion) is located just below the jugular foramen (SECTION VIII.D), as a fusiform swelling of the vagus trunk. It supplies parasympathetic innervation to the pharynx, larynx, trachea, bronchi, esophagus and other viscera. The superior vagal ganglion, located within the foramen about 1cm above it, conveys sensory input from the skin of the ear and from the intracranial meninges.

The solitary tract nucleus is located in the medulla anterior and extending inferior to the dorsal vagus nucleus. Thus, it is also anterior to the fourth ventricle. The cell bodies which send their axons into the solitary tract nucleus are located in the inferior vagal ganglion. The solitary tract nucleus receives sensory input from the taste buds of the mucous membranes of the upper pharynx and epiglottis. It receives this input not only from the superior laryngeal vagus branch, but also from the chorda tympani (part of the facial nerve) and glossopharyngeal nerve. From the latter nerve, it also receives bitter and sour taste sensation from the posterior third of the tongue.

The spinal nucleus of the trigeminal (SECTION IV.A.2) also receives sensory input from the vagus nerve, primarily pain and temperature information from the external ear canal and the skin of the posterior external ear, as well as the meninges of the posterior fossa. The vagus cell bodies which extend their axons into this nucleus are largely found in the jugular ganglion. This ganglion is part of both the glossopharyngeal and vagus systems as they pass through the jugular foramen. It receives parasympathetic motor fibers from the inferior salivatory nucleus of the brain and provides secretomotor innervation to the parotid (salivary) glands. It also connects sensory input from the pharyngeal plexus, the tonsils, taste from the posterior one-third of the tongue, the soft palate, the carotid sinus and certain muscles of the neck to the nucleus of the solitary tract (sensory) in the medulla (ILLUSTRATION 1-65).

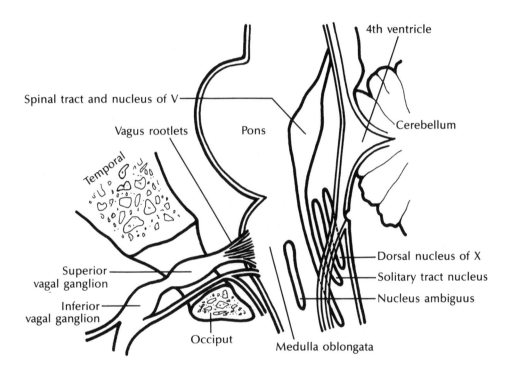

Illustration 1-65
Central Nuclei of the Vagus Nerve (X)

The nucleus ambiguus is composed of motor nerve cells located (bilaterally) entirely within the reticular formation as it passes through the medulla. This nucleus is anterior to the spinal nucleus and tract of the trigeminal. Its motor fibers travel within the glossopharyngeal and accessory systems as well as the vagus system, and supply voluntary muscles of the soft palate, larynx and pharynx. The connection between these muscles, the three cranial nerves, the nucleus ambiguus and the reticular (alarm) system may explain why we shout or scream so readily when our reticular system is activated.

C. Vagus nerve within the cranial cavity

The nerve trunk formed by the union of the vagus rootlets is rather flat and wide. It passes beneath the flocculus of the cerebellum. From its origin, the vagus nerve trunk goes anteriorly and laterally, directly to the jugular foramen, a distance of 2-3cm. Within the cranial cavity, the vagus trunk lies within the subarachnoid space and is closely paralleled by the accessory nerve. The two nerves enter the anterior part of the jugular foramen, taking a common sheath of dura mater with them (ILLUSTRATION 1-66). The glossopharyngeal nerve is separated from the other two nerves by a fibrous band which crosses the foramen; it also has a separate dural sheath.

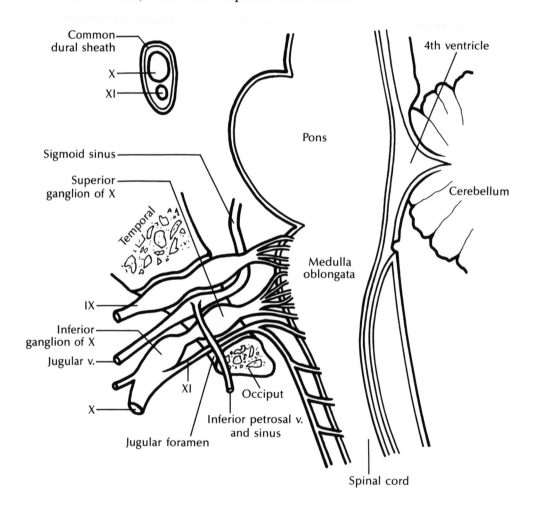

Illustration 1-66
Glossopharyngeal (IX), Vagus (X) and
Accessory (XI) Nerves in the Jugular Foramen

The sigmoid venous sinus (distal end) enters the jugular foramen behind the vagus and accessory nerves, and forms the superior bulb of the internal jugular vein within the foramen. The inferior petrosal venous sinus enters the anterior part of the foramen in front of the cranial nerves, and empties into the same superior bulb (ILLUSTRATION 1-66). Thus, within the foramen the three cranial nerves are at the mercy of venous outflow from within the skull and back pressure from below. Obviously, vasodilation due to venous back pressure may compromise function of these nerves. Since the foramen is essentially a widening of the suture between the occiput and the petrous temporal, it is also apparent that occipito-temporal dysfunction can influence both venous drainage from within the skull and cranial nerve function.

Within the jugular foramen, the vagus nerve enlarges to form the superior vagal ganglion, which is less than 6mm in diameter. The meningeal branches from this ganglion travel back up the vagus into the cranial cavity to distribute to the meninges of the posterior fossa. There is also an auricular branch which enters the ganglion from the skin of the ear canal and the posterior surface of the external ear. This nerve travels to the superior ganglion via the mastoid caniculus which opens into the lateral wall of the foramen.

There are also communications between the superior vagal ganglion and the accessory nerve, the inferior ganglion of the glossopharyngeal nerve, the facial nerve and the jugular sympathetic nerve which extends up from the superior cervical sympathetic ganglion. After all these communications, the vagus passes uneventfully out of the jugular foramen, between the glossopharyngeal and accessory nerves.

Within the foramen, the vagus nerve receives motor fibers from the accessory nerve system. Peripherally, the vagus delivers these fibers to the voluntary muscles of the soft palate, pharynx, larynx and epiglottis.

D. Vagus nerve beyond the jugular foramen in the neck

Inferior to its exit from the jugular foramen, the vagus nerve enlarges to form the inferior vagal ganglion. Afferent fibers coming into this ganglion from the periphery provide input from the many respiratory, digestive and circulatory organs served by the vagus system. The location of this ganglion helps explain the far-reaching effects of the occipital-cranial base release technique.

At the inferior vagal ganglion, there is communication with the glossopharyngeal nerve, accessory nerve, cervical sympathetic trunks and the roots of C1 and C2. Sometimes there is also a branch of the carotid sinus nerve from the ganglion which co-innervates that sinus in conjunction with the glossopharyngeal nerve.

Below the ganglion, the vagus nerve travels vertically downward through the neck within the carotid sheath. Inside the sheath, the vagus lies between the internal jugular vein and internal carotid artery. The vagus is within the sheath throughout the neck, and therefore anterior to the prevertebral fascia (CHAPTER 2). The phrenic nerve is external to the carotid sheath so that factors which affect one of these two nerves do not often affect the other.

The vagus branches repeatedly within the neck. As mentioned, the meningeal and auricular branches arise within the jugular foramen. At the upper part of the inferior vagal ganglion, there are usually two pharyngeal branches contributing to the plexus which supplies both sensory and motor innervation to the soft palate and pharynx. Also, fibers from the pharyngeal branches contribute to the carotid plexuses which supply the carotid sinus and carotid body (SECTION VII.D). These pharyngeal branches pass across the lateral side of the internal carotid artery from the inferior ganglion in order to get to the plexus, located on the superior border of the superior pharyngeal constrictor muscles.

The next branch to arise from the vagus as it runs downward through the neck is the superior laryngeal nerve, which emerges just below the inferior ganglion. This nerve communicates with the superior cervical sympathetic ganglion as it descends down the neck behind the internal carotid artery. At about the level of the carotid bifurcation, this nerve divides into external and internal branches. The external branch travels downward along the side of the larynx under the sternothyroid muscle, along with the superior thyroid artery. It gives motor innervation to the cricothyroid muscles and part of the inferior pharyngeal constrictor muscles and usually contributes to the pharyngeal plexus. The internal branch is larger than the external. It curves forward on the thyrohyoid membrane, pierces the membrane in company with the superior laryngeal artery and enters the larynx, where it supplies sensory innervation to the mucous membrane and parasympathetic secretory/motor innervation to the glands in the epiglottis, base of the tongue and larynx. A terminal fiber communicates with the recurrent laryngeal nerve (see below).

Next, two or three superior cervical cardiac branches emerge from the descending vagus to communicate with cervical sympathetic nerves. The levels at which these branches arise is variable. There are also a few branches (referred to as the inferior cardiac branches) which arise in the lower part of the neck. The lowest of these comes off the vagus just above the first rib. On the right side, these inferior cervical cardiac nerves join the deep cardiac nerve plexus. On the left side, the nerves pass over the arch of the aorta and join the superficial cardiac plexus.

These cardiac branches all communicate and intertwine with sympathetic nerves and glossopharyngeal nerve branches to form the plexuses which innervate the carotid sinuses, carotid bodies and heart. Is it any wonder that good manipulative treatment to the neck can have such positive effects upon blood pressure, heart function and breathing activity?

The recurrent laryngeal nerves are the last major branches of the vagus before it enters the thorax. The right recurrent laryngeal nerve arises from the right vagus nerve as it passes in front of the subclavian artery, loops under and behind the artery and then ascends along the right side of the trachea and esophagus. The left recurrent actually branches from the vagus after the nerve has entered the thorax, just before it passes over the arch of the aorta, loops under the arch and ascends along the left side of the trachea and esophagus.

Both these recurrent nerves lie deep to the common carotid arteries, and pass beneath the lobes of the thyroid gland. Thus, a thyroid tumor may interfere with speech, and a surgeon who removes the thyroid must be careful not to injure the nerves. The nerves also come in close contact with the inferior thyroid arteries and pass under the lower borders of the inferior pharyngeal constrictor muscles. They then penetrate the cricothyroid membranes deep to the joints between the inferior cornua of the thyroid cartilage and the cricoid cartilage. After entering the larynx, the nerves supply motor innervation to all the laryngeal muscles except the cricothyroid; they are essential for our speech ability.

During their ascent, the recurrent laryngeal nerves give rise to various branches which enter the cardiac plexus; receive sensory input from the mucous membranes of the trachea and esophagus, and provide motor control to the intrinsic muscles of those organs; and supply motor and proprioceptive innervation to the inferior pharyngeal constrictor muscles.

E. Vagus nerve in the thorax

Within the thorax, the two halves of the vagus nerve must be described separately because of the asymmetry of the structures supplied (ILLUSTRATION 1-67).

The right vagus nerve enters the thorax after crossing in front of the right subclavian artery. It then passes downward and backward beside the trachea, behind the right innominate vein, behind the inferior vena cava, behind the right main bronchus and to the esophagus. We will leave the right vagus temporarily as it approaches the esophagus.

The left vagus nerve, after entering the thorax, crosses in front of the aortic arch (the left recurrent laryngeal nerve arises in this area), behind and to the left of the left brachiocephalic vein (it is crossed by the left phrenic nerve in this area), in front of the left subclavian artery as it branches off the aorta, behind the left superior intercostal vein, between the aorta and left pulmonary artery, behind the left main bronchus and toward the esophagus.

Inferior cardiac branches arise from the right vagus and from the right recurrent laryngeal nerve as they lie next to the trachea. On the left side, the inferior cardiac branches arise only from the recurrent laryngeal nerve. These branches end in the deep cardiac plexus. All of the motor fibers supplied to the cardiac plexus from the vagus nerves are preganglionic; the synapses are located within the heart muscle. The axons of these cells then travel to innervate the conduction system of the heart, and the heart muscle itself.

There are also sensory fibers which travel with these vagal cardiac nerves to reach the central nervous system. Their sensory receptors are located in the heart muscle and in the arteries related to the heart, as well as the aorta and perhaps its major arterial branches. Within the aorta, there are also receptors similar to those in the carotid bodies. These receptors give information on oxygen content, carbon dioxide content and acidity/alkalinity (pH) of the blood.

As the vagus trunks descend behind the lungs, they give off branches to the anterior pulmonary plexus, as well as branches which connect with sympathetic nerve fibers to contribute to the posterior pulmonary plexuses. The branches of these plexuses follow the bronchi and bronchioles. The posterior pulmonary plexus freely interacts with cardiac, aortic and esophageal plexuses. It is this plexus which acts to contract the bronchiolar muscles and produces the respiratory distress so familiar to people with asthma and other breathing problems.

After passing the roots of the lungs on both sides, the vagus nerve trunks usually divide into two, three or four main trunks as they approach the esophagus. Here the contribute to the esophageal plexus which also receives contributions from the splanchnic nerves and the sympathetic nerve chains. As the vagus trunks descend on the esophagus, they are embedded in the adventitial tissue of its outer wall. The left vagus bundles begin to cover the anterior wall of the esophagus and the right vagus bundles move posteriorly, as though the esophagus was rotated clockwise (looking down from above) with the vagus nerves remaining in constant relationship to it.

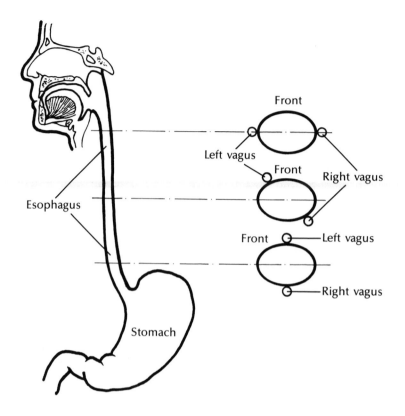

Illustration 1-67
Sections Showing Rotations of Right and Left
Vagus Nerves as They Descend Through the Thorax

Just above the diaphragm there is an intermingling of fibers between the left and right vagus bundles as they descend within the esophageal wall. The bundles on the anterior esophageal wall unite to form a single nerve trunk, as do those on the posterior wall. As a result, the vagus nerve system passes through the esophageal hiatus in the diaphragm as anterior and posterior vagus nerves. Both of these newly formed trunks contain fibers from what were formerly the right and left vagus nerves of the upper thorax.

F. Vagus nerve below the diaphragm

Within the abdomen, these two trunks carry both parasympathetic motor and visceral sensory fibers. They innervate the stomach, pylorus, liver, gall bladder, bile ducts, pancreas and duodenum. The terminal branch of the posterior vagus enters the celiac plexus and contributes to the innervation of the kidneys, spleen, small intestine and the large intestine between its origin in the lower right quadrant of the abdomen and the splenic flexure in the upper left quadrant.

G. Clinical picture

The vagus system is indeed a complex one, with many target organs. It is probably a false separation to divide it from the glossopharyngeal and accessory nerve systems, but scientists love to fragment things for purposes of study. Nevertheless, you can easily see the clinical effects that disturbance of any of these three cranial nerve systems can produce. You can see why jugular foramen dysfunction can be the underlying problem in heart palpitations, digestive disorders, bowel problems, etc. In other words, it is no exaggeration to say that cranial dysfunction can reach down into your bowels and sacral dysfunction can reach up into your heart. Any part of the craniosacral system can contribute to jugular foramen dysfunction, which can in turn affect the vagus nerve system and any or all of its target organs.

IX. ACCESSORY NERVE

I have, of necessity, said a lot about the accessory nerve (XI) during the preceding discussions of the glossopharyngeal and vagus nerves (SECTIONS VII and VIII). The accessory nerve is perhaps most easily thought of as the inferior end of the cranial nerve IX/X/XI complex. There is considerable interaction, shared anatomy and functional overlap among the three nerves.

The accessory nerve is a motor nerve and consists of a spinal part and a cranial part. The spinal part is derived from a variable number of upper cervical spinal nerve roots. Usually, it is about the upper five cervical segments which produce motor roots contributing to the formation of the spinal part of the accessory nerve. The cranial part is integrated with the vagus nerve in terms of its central nuclei and peripheral distribution (ILLUSTRATION 1-68).

A. Spinal part of the accessory nerve

Let's look first at the course of the spinal part. It is derived from the upper spinal motor roots in the cervical region. These motor roots are made up of axons of motor cells located in the lateral ventral columns of the gray matter in the spinal cord. The cells are arranged in a column on each side of the cord. We call them the spinal nuclei of the accessory nerve. Each nucleus is (perhaps) an extension of the visceral efferent column that extends down from the medulla. The motor roots exit the spinal cord laterally about halfway between the ventral and dorsal roots, ascend under cover of the dura mater and join the root above until all five roots are united into a common trunk. This trunk is called the spinal accessory nerve. The trunk ascends bilaterally and passes through the foramen magnum behind the vertebral artery. Inside the skull, the nerve trunk crosses the occiput in the subarachnoid space, is joined by the cranial accessory nerve and exits though the jugular foramen.

B. Cranial part of the accessory nerve

The cranial part of the accessory nerve is actually an accessory to the vagus nerve and is more realistically considered in that context. The central nucleus of the cranial

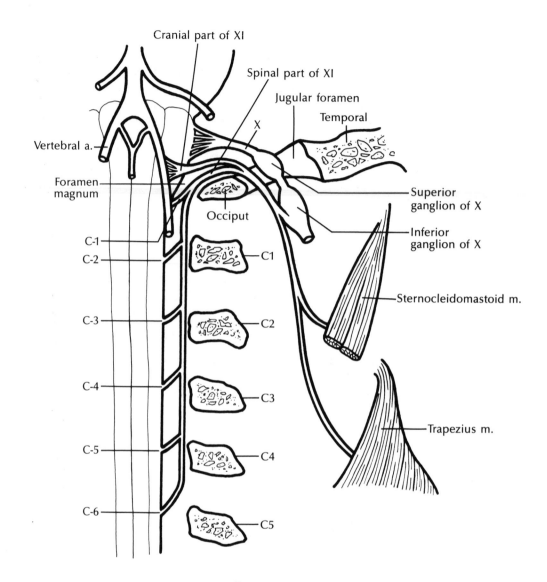

Illustration 1-68
Accessory Nerve (XI)

part is the inferior part of the nucleus ambiguus which also serves the vagus and glossopharyngeal nerves (SECTION VIII.B). It may also receive minor contributions from the dorsal vagal nucleus. There are four or five pair of cranial accessory rootlets exiting the medulla; they are in series with (and below) the rootlets of the vagal and glossopharyngeal nerves (SECTION VIII.A). They join to form the cranial accessory trunk, which runs laterally in the subdural space, joins the spinal trunk (which is significantly larger) and enters the jugular foramen. As the cranial rootlets leave the medulla, they come into a variable relationship with the posterior inferior cerebellar artery (SECTION VII.B).

C. Union and separation

Within the jugular foramen, the cranial accessory trunk exchanges some fibers with the spinal trunk; there is also communication with the superior vagal ganglion. Immediately after exiting the skull through the foramen, the spinal and cranial trunks separate again. The cranial part blends with the vagus nerve upon which it relies for distribution of its motor innervation to the uvula, levator veli palatini, pharyngeal constrictor muscle and muscles of the larynx and esophagus. Actually, the cranial accessory trunk has no peripheral nerves which are exclusively its own after it separates from the spinal part.

The spinal trunk is exclusively voluntary motor in function. It innervates the sternocleidomastoid and trapezius muscles. After exiting the jugular foramen, it turns backward, passing behind, in front of or through the internal jugular vein. It then goes behind the stylohyoid and digastric muscles to the sternocleidomastoid and trapezius. En route, it passes through the posterior triangle of the neck where it is covered only by fascia.

Dysfunction of the jugular foramen may cause contraction of the sternocleidomastoid or trapezius via the accessory system, which can then further aggravate the jugular foramen dysfunction. A "vicious circle" is thereby set in motion which in turn can affect the glossopharyngeal and vagus systems, and elevate venous back pressure within the cranial vault.

After exiting the jugular foramen, the spinal accessory trunk communicates with spinal segments C2, C3 and C4. This is probably to provide proprioceptive input to the system, but also provides potential for further self-perpetuation of the vicious circle mentioned above.

X. HYPOGLOSSAL NERVE

The hypoglossal nerve (XII) is a motor nerve supplying the muscles of the tongue.

A. Central nuclei

The central nuclei of the hypoglossal system are columns of cells about 2cm long lying on each side of the medulla, close to the midline in the gray matter. Each nucleus receives fibers from the cortex through the corticobulbar tracts. Some are from the same side, but most are crossed. These nuclei also communicate with cortical centers (via the extrapyramidal and tectobulbar tracts), the hypothalamic visceral centers, and the trigeminal, glossopharyngeal and vagal sensory nuclei in the pons and medulla. These interconnections reflect the varied functions of the tongue.

B. Intracranial course of the hypoglossal nerve

The axons of the motor cells of the hypoglossal nucleus exit from the medulla in a series of rootlets, the number of which is variable up to perhaps eight on each side. After exiting the medulla, the rootlets are gathered together into two bundles on each side. This gathering occurs in the subarachnoid space. The two pair of bundles perforate the dura mater separately, pass behind the vertebral artery, pass through hypoglossal canals in the occipital bone and finally unite. In some cases, each canal is divided by a bony spicule, giving each hypoglossal bundle its own canal. The internal entrances of the canals are high in the foramen magnum above the occipital condyles; the exits are just lateral to the condyles.

C. Union and separation

As it emerges bilaterally from the canal, the nerve is behind the internal carotid artery and the internal jugular vein and posterior/medial to the glossopharyngeal, vagus and accessory nerves. It runs downward, adhering closely to the vagus nerve with which it communicates. It also communicates with the sympathetic nerves and (chiefly) with the inferior vagal ganglion (ILLUSTRATION 1-69).

The hypoglossal nerve travels deep to the digastric muscle and occipital artery, anterior to the external carotid artery, lingual nerve and middle pharyngeal constrictor muscles, above the greater cornu of the hyoid, forward and upward over the hyoglossus and genioglossus muscles, deep to the central digastric tendon, stylohyoid and mylohyoid muscles and inferior to the submandibular glands. The end branches of the nerve go upward into the tongue and forward into the top of the tongue by communicating with the lingual and glossopharyngeal nerves.

After exiting the hypoglossal canal, the nerve communicates with the superior cervical sympathetic ganglion, inferior vagal ganglion, pharyngeal plexus, lingual nerve (near the hyoglossus muscle) and C1/C2, which supply the supra- and infrahyoid muscles.

Some authors describe tiny filaments given off in the hypoglossal canals which go back to the dura mater as sensory innervation (HOLLINGSHEAD 1968). This is probably a case of other sensory nerves "hitching a ride" with the hypoglossal nerve.

As the hypoglossal nerve loops around the occipital artery deeply to the digastric muscle, it gives off a branch called the superior root of the ansa cervicalis. The origin of the fibers in this root are from the communication with the roots of C1. They are not from the hypoglossal nucleus. This nerve travels on the surface of the carotid sheath to the middle cervical level, innervates the superior belly of the omohyoid muscle and then becomes the medial arm of the ansa cervicalis loop. The lateral arm of this loop is derived from C2 and C3; its nerve branches supply the inferior belly of the omohyoid muscle, the sternohyoid muscle and the sternothyroid muscle. There are also C1 fibers to the thyrohyoid and geniohyoid muscles which travel within the hypoglossal trunk.

True hypoglossal nerve fibers which arise from the hypoglossal nucleus go only to the intrinsic muscles of the tongue and to the styloglossus, hyoglossus, genioglossus and chrondroglossus muscles.

It is the relationship of the hypoglossal nerve to the occipital condyles which is of greatest interest to the craniosacral therapist. Dysfunction or compression of the condyles can easily influence hypoglossal nerve function, which is manifested as impaired tongue movement. Release of the cranial base and condyles is always indicated in cases where tongue movement is abnormal or impaired.

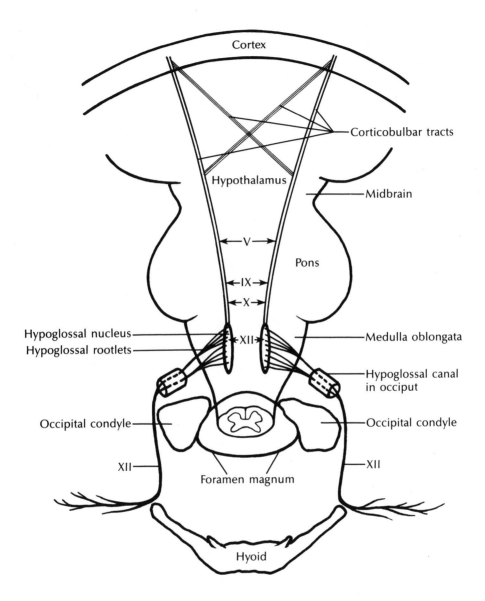

Illustration 1-69
Hypoglossal Nerve (XII)

XI. CRANIAL NERVES: SUMMARY

We have spent a lot of time discussing the anatomy and physiology of the cranial nerves, and how they relate to the craniosacral system of diagnosis and treatment. I know of no better way to defeat the purpose of this presentation than to leave it in a complex, highly detailed and fragmented condition. This is especially true for those practitioners who focus upon the very subtle physiological motions, responses and energies upon which craniosacral therapy is based. Craniosacral therapy is both a highly intuitive art form and a highly scientific modality. It is not my intent to disturb this balance, so in summary let us look at the cranial nerve system in a quick overview.

The petrous temporal bone affords passage to the facial and vestibulocochlear nerves. We can use the petrous temporal bone as a dividing line. All cranial nerves ahead of the facial nerve (VII) in the numbering sequence are most likely to be affected by dysfunction of the anterior half of the cranial base. That is, cranial nerves I through VI will most likely become dysfunctional in conjunction with somatic dysfunctions involving the fronto-ethmoidal complex, the sphenoid and temporal bones.

Problems with cranial nerves VII and VIII will generally be related to temporal bone dysfunction, whereas problems with nerves IX through XI will more likely relate to the temporo-occipital suture and jugular foramen. Dysfunction of the hypoglossal nerve (XII) will probably be secondary to problems of the occipital condyles and the atlanto-occipital joint.

In terms of membranes, keep in mind that the visual motor nerves (III, IV and VI) pass between the layers of the tentorium cerebelli. Therefore, abnormal tension patterns in this membrane often underlie strabismus. Remember also that cranial nerves usually carry dural sleeves with them for some distance. It is therefore essential that the membrane system be free of abnormal tension.

2.

ANATOMY OF THE NECK

CHAPTER 2

I. INTRODUCTION

The anatomy of the human neck has been dissected and resected and cussed and discussed by students of its architecture for generations. The fasciae of the neck have been presented by authors in many different ways. Each presentation is an attempt to simplify and make the subject more comprehensible according to that author's particular inclination. To the student, it may seem that most of these attempts at simplification have been in vain.

The anatomy of the human neck is indeed complex. In this chapter, I shall attempt to describe this anatomy, integrate structure with function and then discuss the significance of this functional anatomy for the practitioner of craniosacral therapy. I shall try not to get bogged down with detail at the expense of the total view. However, please realize that some detail is required for an understanding of the neck and what it does for its owner.

The human neck does many things. It attaches the head to the body, and therefore serves as a conduit for all nerve impulses passing in either direction. Since the head is the major intelligence gathering and decision-making center for the whole person (though I have met some apparent exceptions), the number of nerve impulses passing through the neck is enormous. Your head is home to most of your sensory organs; the receptors for vision, hearing, equilibrium, smell and taste are all located here. In order to better serve these senses, your head must be able to move in relationship to your body; it is your neck that provides you this service. It is true that touch, proprioception, pain, etc., are perceived in other parts of the body and some simple reflexes are mediated via the spinal cord, but the information always goes through the neck to the head for central integration and decision-making.

All food, drink and air normally reach the body via the head and neck. Blood passes from the body through the neck in order to nourish, protect and remove waste products from the head. Therefore, brain function, sensory system and body activity are all dependent upon the efficient and well-regulated function of transport systems in the neck.

In order to carry out all of these vital and complex activities, the neck must be able to rotate right and left, side-bend in both directions, flex (forward) and extend (backward). It must also support the weight of the head and not interfere with nerve conduction either inside or outside of the spinal cord; avoid compressing blood and lymph vessels as they pass through; maintain an open air passage; and it must open and close the correct tubes so that food and drink may be properly swallowed. Because of its ability to perform this multiplicity of functions, the neck represents a masterpiece of anatomical "engineering."

In discussing the neck in the context of craniosacral therapy, we will be concerned primarily with fasciae, cartilage, the hyoid bone and muscles, and to a lesser extent with associated nerves, vessels, glands and other structures.

II. CERVICAL FASCIAE

A. Introduction

The cervical fasciae provide support and compartmentalization for all of the other structures of the neck. Once you have a clear comprehension of these fasciae, the remaining tissues and their functions are much easier to understand.

The cervical fasciae may be viewed as tubes within tubes. These tubes are oriented longitudinally so that they serve to connect head to body. The walls of the tubes separate at appropriate times to provide compartments or envelopes which accommodate the other structures of the neck. Separate compartments or envelopes of fascia are provided for all bones, muscles, visceral organs (such as the thyroid gland, esophagus and trachea), nerves and vessels. In craniosacral therapy, we must consider and appreciate the effect which these fascial tubes and compartments have upon the vitality and function of the tissues which they surround.

B. Cervical meninges

First, let us examine the fascial tubes which are located within the vertebral canal of the neck. These tubes, the cervical meninges, are of particular interest to craniosacral therapists. They constitute the cervical portion of Sutherland's "core link" (i.e., the tube of dura mater as it functionally and structurally connects the occiput with the sacrum).

We will look at the fasciae of the neck from the inside out. The spinal cord will be used as our central reference point.

1. Background. The cervical spinal cord serves as the major conductor of nerve impulses between the brain and the spinal cord below the neck. The spinal cord, of course, ultimately connects the brain with the peripheral nervous system. There are a few nerve pathways external to the spinal cord which serve the same function, among them the sympathetic nerve chains whose fibers enter the skull in association with arteries, as well as with the glossopharyngeal, vagus and accessory cranial nerves (CHAPTER 1, SECTIONS VII-IX).

The medulla oblongata, the most caudal part of the brain, is continuous with the cervical spinal cord at the level of the foramen magnum (the large opening in the occiput where it sits on top of the spinal column). The cervical spinal cord gives off eight pair of dorsal and ventral roots. Each side of each spinal cord segment gives off one dorsal and one ventral root which unite temporarily to form a common trunk somewhere within the intervertebral foramen. The dorsal root carries sensory input into the spinal cord from the periphery; the ventral root sends motor commands out to the body from the central nervous system. Of interest at this point is the fact that the ventral motor fibers, after exiting the intervertebral foramen, communicate with the sympathetic nervous system (SEE "SYMPATHETIC NERVOUS SYSTEM" IN GLOSSARY).

Spinal nerve C1 (called the suboccipital nerve) exits from the vertebral canal between the occiput and the atlas, passes above the arch of the atlas and below the vertebral artery, enters the suboccipital triangle and provides innervation to the muscles which form the triangle (the oblique superior and inferior and the rectus capitis posterior major), as well as the rectus capitis posterior minor and the semispinalis capitis. Occasionally the suboccipital nerve gives off a sensory branch supplying part of the scalp. When present, this branch accompanies the occipital artery and communicates with the greater and lesser occipital nerves, both of which are derived from the roots of C2.

Compression of the occipital condyles and/or occipito-atlal dysfunction secondary to suboccipital muscle hypertonicity can cause dysfunction and facilitation of the suboccipital nerve. Clinically, this relates to the tension headache syndrome at the back of the head, which frequently broadcasts to the frontal region. This syndrome may be effectively treated by the cranial base release technique (UPLEDGER 1983:57).

The greater occipital nerve is largely sensory and enters the vertebral canal from the periphery by passing between the lower surface of the arch of the atlas and the upper surface of the lamina of the axis. This nerve is a major contributor to the dorsal root of C2. It brings in sensory information from the scalp of the back of the head from as high as the vertex. It also services the obliquus capitis inferior muscle and may communicate with the suboccipital nerve.

The lesser occipital nerve is largely motor in function. It is derived from the ventral root of C2, and contributes (along with the ventral [motor] divisions of C1, C3 and C4, and cranial nerves IX, X and XI) to the cervical plexus. The lower five cervical spinal cord segments contribute to the brachial plexus, which innervates the upper extremity.

2. Pia mater. This is the innermost of the three meninges. It closely invests the entire central nervous system and carries the blood vessels which supply nutrients to and remove waste metabolites from the nerve tissue. The pia mater is made up largely of collagen and elastic fibers covered by flattened squamous cells. There are astrocyte projections from the central nervous system which enter the pia mater and penetrate its capillary network, serving to attach the pia mater to the nervous tissue and probably functioning in the selective transportation of ions and molecules into and out of the central nervous system (i.e., as part of the blood-brain barrier).

As each nerve root leaves or enters the spinal cord, the pia mater forms an investing sheath which follows the nerve root as far as the intervertebral foramen. Beyond this foramen, the pia mater sleeve blends with the perineurium of the nerve.

The external surface of the pia mater is intermittently attached to the internal surface of the arachnoid membrane (the second of the three meninges) by fine fibrous trabeculae. The space between the pia mater and arachnoid, appropriately called the subarachnoid space, is filled with cerebrospinal fluid.

The arachnoid also contributes to the sleeve which follows each nerve root to the intervertebral foramen. However, it fuses with the periosteum at the foramen and ends at that point. The subarachnoid space with its contained cerebrospinal fluid also follows each nerve root to the intervertebral foramen, where it ends by fusion of the meningeal layers.

In the cervical spinal area, the pia mater is somewhat thicker and less vascular than it is in the cranium. Anteriorly, it follows and lines the longitudinal ventral fissure of the spinal cord, where it forms a fibrous band called the linea splendens.

The denticulate ligaments, also derived from the pia mater, emerge intersegmentally between the cord roots. They are oriented longitudinally between the dorsal and ventral roots, and form lateral triangular projections which pierce the arachnoid and attach to the inner surface of the dura mater, helping to hold the spinal cord in place (ILLUSTRATION 2-1). There are 21 pair of denticulate ligaments. The uppermost pair attaches to the dura mater at the foramen magnum after passing between the vertebral artery and the hypoglossal nerve. The lowest pair emerges at the T12/L1 junction.

3. Arachnoid. This meningeal membrane is very delicate, much like cellophane paper in appearance under normal conditions, and essentially non-vascular. I have seen

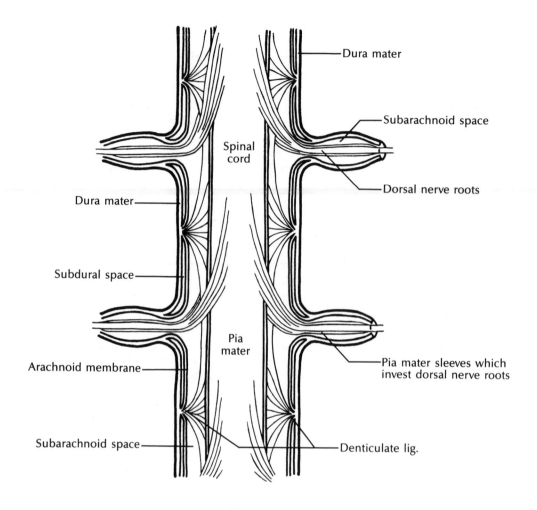

Illustration 2-1
Posterior Cutaway View of the Spinal Cord

edematous arachnoid membranes which appeared to be over 6mm thick due to swelling and fluid retention. The arachnoid is separated from the pia mater by the subarachnoid space, and from the dura mater (the outermost meningeal membrane) by the subdural space. Both of these spaces contain fluid and permit movement between the meningeal layers.

The subarachnoid space contains cerebrospinal fluid (the same fluid found in the ventricles of the brain). Despite close biochemical similarities, there is some disagreement as to whether the fluid in the subdural space may correctly be called cerebrospinal fluid. I believe it can; however, from a practical point of view in the context of craniosacral therapy, it makes little or no difference what we call it.

Inside the skull the arachnoid does not follow the pia mater into all the little fissures and sulci of the brain, except where it follows the falxes and the tentorium as these membranes make their entrance between the hemispheres of the cerebrum and the cerebellum, and thereby helps to separate the two halves of the brain.

Within the vertebral canal, the arachnoid is a tubular sheath which loosely encloses the pia mater and its contents, the spinal cord and the spinal nerve roots. The cervical arachnoid is, of course, continuous with the intracranial arachnoid above and the thoracic arachnoid below. Throughout the length of the spinal cord, the arachnoid invests all the nerve roots, including the cauda equina into which the cord terminates inferiorly.

The subdural space is smaller in volume under normal conditions than is the subarachnoid space. The arachnoid does not connect to the dura mater as it does to the pia mater by its trabeculations. Arachnoid-dural connections occur only at their common mooring sites, such as the intervertebral foramina where both membranes terminate after sheathing the nerve roots.

4. Dura mater. Within the cranial vault, there are two layers of the dura mater, closely connected by trabeculae. After passing through the foramen magnum into the cervical vertebral canal, these two layers become almost totally separated and independent of each other. The outer layer, which in the skull is the endosteum (internal periosteum) of the skull bones, continues into the cervical canal as the periosteum of the cervical vertebrae and as the lining of the vertebral canal. The inner layer becomes the spinal dura mater, and loosely invests the spinal cord. In the cervical region, the spinal dura begins at the foramen magnum (to which it is very firmly attached around the circumference) and descends through the vertebral canal with minimal attachment to other fasciae and bones. It forms loose sheaths which accompany the spinal nerve roots as they exit the spinal cord. These sheaths, like those of the arachnoid, terminate at the intervertebral foramina.

These dural attachments cannot be regarded as being within the vertebral canal; within the canal, the dura moves with relative independence from the arachnoid and from the vertebrae. The restricting moorings for the spinal dura are limited to the foramen magnum, C2, C3 and S2. This arrangement allows for relatively unencumbered movement of the spinal cord within the vertebral canal; otherwise, we would stretch and stress our spinal cords as we move our necks and backs.

The space between the spinal dura and the inner periosteum of the vertebrae (formerly the two intracranial layers of dura mater) is called the epidural cavity (or space). This cavity contains a quantity of loose areolar tissue and a venous plexus (analogous to the venous sinus system in the skull), and facilitates movement between the spinal dura and the lining of the canal.

The spinal dura attaches to the foramen magnum and to the posterior bodies of C2 and C3. Clinically, this means that problems affecting dural mobility within the vertebral canal will frequently manifest as upper cervical spinal dysfunction and as occipital problems with severe pain. The spinal dura connects by fibrous slips to the posterior longitudinal ligament; however, this ligament does not restrict the dural tube as much as the attachments at C2, C3 and S2 (ILLUSTRATION 2-2).

I have seen many examples of coccygeal injury which related etiologically to upper cervical and/or head pain. I have just finished treating (successfully) a 28-year-old woman whose headaches were relieved by functional correction of a spinal somatic dysfunction at the thoracolumbar junction. The latter injury preceded the onset of headaches by about a year. It resulted from a hyperextension strain sustained during a gymnastic workout.

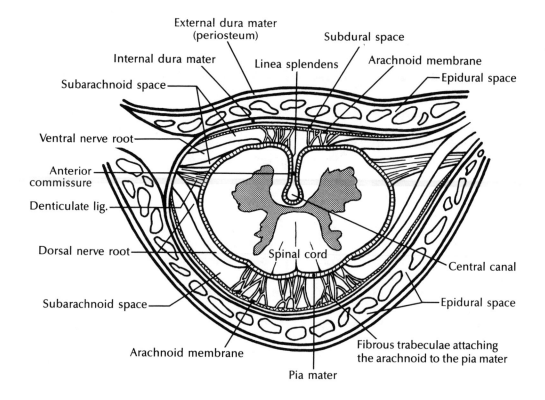

Illustration 2-2
Cross Section of the Cervical Spine

Yet another example of head/neck pain due to dysfunction/injury to the lower spine is that of an 8-year-old girl who sustained upper thoracic injury in an auto accident. No fractures were found using diagnostic imagery. Within weeks of the accident she developed constant frontal head pain and some cerebral dysfunction manifested by a decline in academic performance and confirmed by a psychologist. Cranial dysfunction was predominantly a frontal bone retraction into compression, apparently caused by membrane hypertonus. Correction of the upper thoracic problem using functional release technique resulted in spontaneous release of the frontal bone dysfunction with immediate alleviation of head pain and a more gradual improvement in academic performance.

The lumbar epidural space was commonly used in the 1960's for the deposition of anesthetic agents during childbirth. The result was the reduction of pain sensation during contractions, with minimal reduction of the force of contraction. This technique is less popular today because of a variety of possible complications.

C. Prevertebral fascia

The use of the prefix "pre-" attached to the word "vertebral" in this phrase can be misleading. Many students justifiably understand this to mean that the prevertebral fascia is located anterior to the vertebrae. Actually, the prevertebral fascia forms a vertically oriented cylinder of connective tissue which almost completely encircles the vertebral column and its related soft tissues.

1. Attachments. Posteriorly, the prevertebral fascia attaches to the nuchal ligament and the spines of the cervical vertebrae. Laterally, it attaches to the anterior tubercles of the cervical transverse processes. It completes its cylindrical shape by covering the anterior aspects of the vertebral bodies. This fascial sheath therefore contains within it the spinal cord, the three layers of meningeal fascia described above, the vertebral column and the posterior, lateral and anterior muscles which are related to the vertebrae. It also contains all of the associated nerves, vessels, muscle sheaths and connective tissue structures.

Superiorly, the prevertebral fascia is attached to the base of the skull, surrounding the attachments of most of the cervical muscles. The fascial cylinder therefore contains all of the muscles which attach to the occiput deep to the trapezius (rectus capitis posterior major/minor, obliquus capitis superior, semispinalis capitis and splenius capitis), as well as the sternocleidomastoid. Superiorly directed traction on the occiput stretches the prevertebral fascia as well as the nuchal ligament and all of its related cervical vertebral spinous processes (ILLUSTRATION 2-3).

As the prevertebral fascial attachment to the skull continues laterally in both directions, it crosses the suture between the occiput and the temporal bone. Here it invests the splenius capitis muscle which attaches to the roughened surfaces of the underside of the skull. It then angles medially behind the jugular fossa and the carotid canal, and attaches loosely to the carotid sheath which invests the structures passing through these openings. It then follows the suture line between the occiput and petrous temporal antero-medially so that the fascial sheath encloses the occipital condyles and the rectus capitis lateralis muscles laterally and the longis capitis and rectus capitis anterior muscles anteriorly. The two lateral sides of the prevertebral fascia turn medially and meet at the midline of the skull just posterior to the sphenobasilar synchondrosis on the occiput. Thus, the attachment of the prevertebral fascia to the skull makes a distorted circle which includes the attachments of the vertebral muscles to the skull as well as the joints which connect the skull to the neck.

The prevertebral fascia descends from its skull attachments to the cervical/thoracic junction, where it extends along the anterior surface of the vertebral musculature into the superior mediastinum of the thorax and becomes continuous with the anterior longitudinal ligament. An anterior lamina of the prevertebral fascia detaches from its posterior sheet and fuses with the esophagus at the level of the angle of Louis (sternum).

2. Relationships to nerves and muscles. As the roots of the brachial plexus emerge from between the anterior and middle scalene muscles in the posterior triangle of the neck, the prevertebral fascia provides a sheath for these nerve roots, and for the subclavian artery, as they run beneath the clavicle into the axilla (armpit). This prolongation becomes the axillary neuromuscular sheath. This continuity of fascia provides the means by which the arm and the neck relate in terms of cause and effect in pain syndromes and dysfunctions.

The posterior triangle of the neck has as its boundaries the sternocleidomastoid muscle in front, the trapezius muscle behind and the middle third of the clavicle as its base. The prevertebral fascia is the floor or deep side of the triangle. In the upper

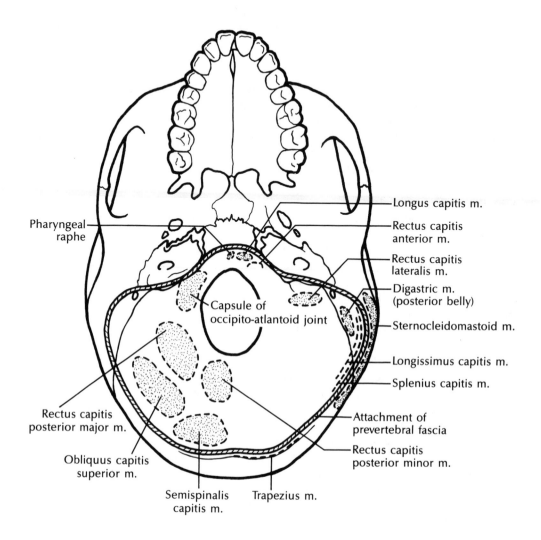

Illustration 2-3
Attachments of Prevertebral Fascia to Skull

part of the triangle, the prevertebral fascia and the superficial fascia are in close contact, being separated only by a cleavage plane. Thus, as the cutaneous branches of the cervical nerve plexus emerge at the posterior border of the sternocleidomastoid muscle, the nerves pierce the two fascial layers almost simultaneously. The accessory nerve crosses the posterior triangle and lies between the two fascial layers (ILLUSTRATION 2-4).

In the lower part of the posterior triangle nearer the clavicle the two fascial layers separate to form a space which is filled with loose connective tissue and fat. Also in this space are the subclavian vein, lower end of the external jugular vein, transverse cervical vessels, suprascapular vessels, supraclavicular vessels and posterior belly of the omohyoid muscle. This space communicates with no other space in the neck, and functions as an obstacle to transmission of infection.

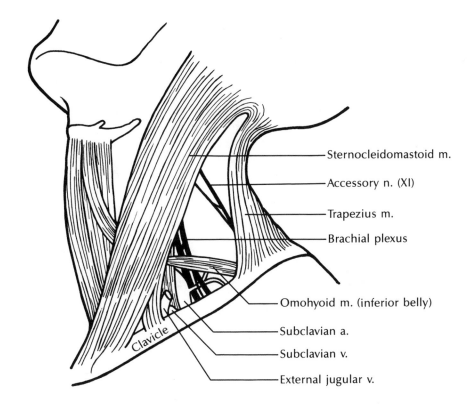

Illustration 2-4
Posterior Triangle of the Neck

Beneath the sternocleidomastoid muscle, the prevertebral and superficial fasciae separate. The superficial fascia then extends anteriorly and laterally to the internal jugular vein and the common carotid artery, and contributes to the anterolateral layer of the carotid sheath. The prevertebral fascia turns medially behind the internal jugular vein, common carotid artery and vagus nerve. In order to allow for independent movement of the vertebral column and its musculature, this fascia is separated from the posterior wall of the carotid sheath by an abundance of loose connective tissue. This part of the prevertebral fascia thus overlies the scalene muscles, and is often called the scalene fascia.

The phrenic nerve, en route from its origin at C4 to its destination at the diaphragm, lies on the anterior surface of the anterior scalene muscle, between the muscle and the prevertebral fascia and under the sternocleidomastoid muscle. It is crossed by the inferior belly of the omohyoid muscle and the transverse cervical and suprascapular vessels, and enters the thorax with the anterior scalene muscle after passing between the subclavian artery and vein.

The brachial plexus passes between the anterior and middle scalene muscles on its way to the arm. The prevertebral fascia forms an axillary sheath investing the plexus and its branches as they service the arm muscles.

The cervical sympathetic nerve trunk is embedded within the prevertebral fascia, running longitudinally just anterior to the fascia's attachment to the cervical transverse processes.

The prevertebral fascia divides into two lamina anteriorly where it separates the esophagus from the anterior musculature of the vertebral column. The anterior and posterior portions are called the alar and prevertebral lamina, respectively. The compartment thus formed begins at the level of the skull and continues downward to the thoracic cavity, and is often referred to as the "danger space" because it provides an avenue for spread of infection between the neck and the thorax. I suspect the purpose of this space is to allow movement between the vertebral column (and its associated structures) and the esophagus and trachea. This lamination of the fasciae provides reasonably friction-free sliding surfaces (ILLUSTRATION 2-5).

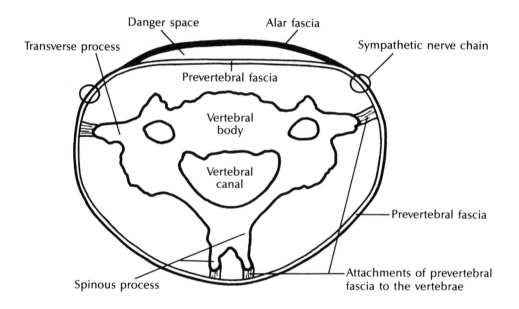

Illustration 2-5
Cross Section of Prevertebral Fascia

D. Pretracheal fascia

The name pretracheal fascia describes the position of this fascia between the hyoid bone and pericardium anterior to the trachea. It contributes to a fascial tube which encircles the trachea and the esophagus; the lateral portions of the tube are contributed by the carotid sheaths, and the posterior portion by the alar lamina of the prevertebral fascia. In addition to blending laterally with the carotid sheaths, the pretracheal fascia connects with the superficial fasciae. A less commonly used term for the pretracheal fascia is "visceral fascia" (ILLUSTRATION 2-6).

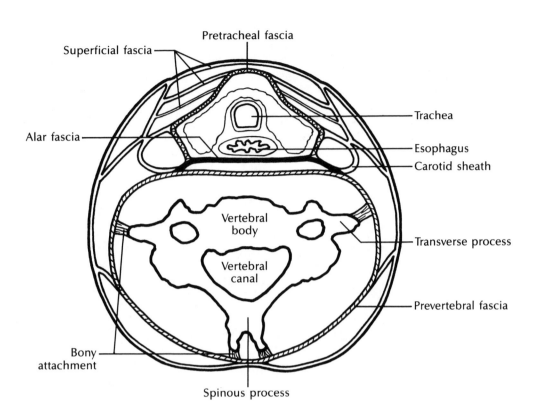

Illustration 2-6
Pretracheal Fascia

In comparison to the prevertebral fascia, the pretracheal fascia is much thinner and more delicate, although the anterior prevertebral fascia is microscopically more dense than is its extension behind the esophagus.

The pretracheal fascia laminae divide to form an envelope which houses the thyroid gland. This envelope actually blends with and contributes to the capsule of the thyroid, and is penetrated by the vessels and nerves which service the gland.

The pretracheal fascia attaches firmly to the thyroid cartilage and the hyoid bone above. Above this hyoid attachment it is continuous with the buccopharyngeal fascia. This latter fascia attaches to the inferior surface of the body of the sphenoid bone, and is continuous bilaterally with the fasciae of the external surfaces of the buccinator muscles. This arrangement provides continuity between the thyroid cartilage, hyoid bone and sphenoid bone.

Below the hyoid bone, the pretracheal fascia travels down the neck behind the infrahyoid (strap) muscles and is ultimately blended with the anterior fibrous pericardium behind the sternum. This arrangement provides continuity between the sphenoid bone and the pericardium. The hyoid bone and the thyroid cartilage are imposed between these two ends of the fascia, much like moveable or floating moorings for the pretracheal and buccopharyngeal fasciae.

E. Carotid sheaths

These are paired, longitudinally-oriented fascial tubes, derived largely from superficial fascia, which pass vertically through the neck, enclosing the common and internal carotid arteries, jugular veins and vagus nerves. The sheaths are located deep to the sternocleidomastoid muscle and blend with the pretracheal fascia anteriorly and the prevertebral fascia medially.

The carotid sheath is divided into three separate compartments. The internal jugular vein is usually anterior and lateral, the vagus nerve posterior to and partially between the artery and the vein and the carotid artery is usually antero-medial to, or directly medial to, the vagus nerve (ILLUSTRATION 2-7).

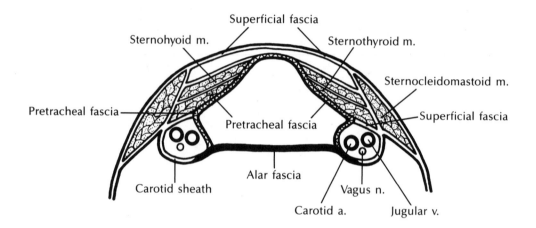

Illustration 2-7
Carotid Sheaths

Above, the carotid sheath attaches directly to the inferior surface of the cranial base, forming an oval around the carotid canal (which pierces the petrous temporal and affords passage to the internal carotid artery) and the jugular foramen (CHAPTER 1).

The carotid sheath provides an opening and a fascial sleeve for the external carotid artery as it branches off from the common carotid artery at the level of the upper border of the thyroid cartilage, and encloses the internal carotid artery above the bifurcation. The sheath extends downward into the thorax to blend with the fascia of the aortic arch on the left and the brachiocephalic artery on the right. These arteries give origin to the two common carotid arteries. Actually, the carotid sheaths may be regarded as extensions of the fibrous pericardium into the neck and upward to the skull. Since the fibrous pericardium is blended with the fascia of the respiratory diaphragm, we have fascial continuity from the temporal bones and the occipital bone to the respiratory diaphragm.

We can speculate about the clinical significance of this functional anatomy. Think about the effect of respiratory diaphragm dysfunction on the craniosacral mechanism, especially upon temporal and occipital bone function. Also think about the effect of this connection upon the jugular foramen and its contents. Structures passing through this foramen, and the related dysfunctions, include: (1) The jugular vein. We believe that anatomical dysfunction at this foramen interferes with optimal venous drainage from the cranial vault; (2) the vagus nerve. Symptoms of vagus system dysfunction include fainting spells, light-headedness, heart palpitations and problems in swallowing, speaking, digestive function, breathing and bowel function; (3) the glossopharyngeal nerve. We don't often notice a dysfunction of this nerve because its major function is to help us taste bitter substances on the posterior one-third of the tongue; it isn't something we miss if we lose it; and (4) the spinal accessory nerve, which is motor to the sternocleidomastoid and trapezius, as well as to a variable number of smaller but no less important neck muscles. Obviously, a problem with the jugular foramen can contribute to dysfunction of the muscles of the neck, which can then further contribute to more jugular foramen dysfunction, and so on (CHAPTER 1, SECTION VII).

I have seen many clinical cases wherein diaphragmatic release (which is often accompanied by emotional release) allows a spontaneous release of the temporal bones, which are often restricted in internal rotation in these cases. When temporal bone function is normalized, any or all of the "vagus nerve symptoms" may be alleviated. Congestion headaches are often the result of jugular foramen dysfunction problems caused partially by temporal bone dysfunction, which may be secondary to respiratory diaphragm restriction.

Because of the temporal connection, dysfunctions originating in the thorax or respiratory diaphragm may even be manifested in or contribute to TMJ syndrome (CHAPTER 3).

F. Superficial fascia

The superficial fascia of the neck is continuous with that of the head and face. The arbitrary boundary between the two regions consists of the inferior border of the mandible in front, a line on each side between the mandibular angles and the tip of the mastoid processes of the temporal bones and an extension of these lines around the back of the head-neck junction to the superior nuchal line on the occiput.

Below, the cervical superficial fascia attaches to the clavicles and sternum where it is continuous with the pectoral/deltoid fasciae. Above the sternum, it separates into separate anterior and posterior layers to form the space of Burns immediately above the suprasternal notch. The platysma muscle, which extends from the mandible to the clavicles, is embedded in the cervical superficial fascia. The muscle fibers are often interwoven with the deeper fibers of the fascia. The space of Burns between the superficial fascia and the deeper fascia of the neck in the anterior regions facilitates the independent movement of the platysma (ILLUSTRATIONS 2-8-A and 2-8-B).

Posteriorly, the cervical superficial fascia arises from the spinous processes of the cervical vertebrae and from the nuchal ligament. It encircles the neck and forms a cylinder or sleeve around the cervical structures. The inner aspect of the superficial fascia and the external aspect of the prevertebral fascia are in contact. The superficial fascia divides into two layers and envelops the trapezius muscle. The spinal accessory nerve (CHAPTER 1, SECTION IX) is located deep to the trapezius and between the superficial and prevertebral fascial sheets. After enveloping the trapezius, the two fascial layers unite to form a single layer which covers the posterior triangles of the neck. The posterior triangle is bounded in front by the posterior border of the sternocleidomastoid, and in back by the anterior border of the trapezius. These two meet at the occiput

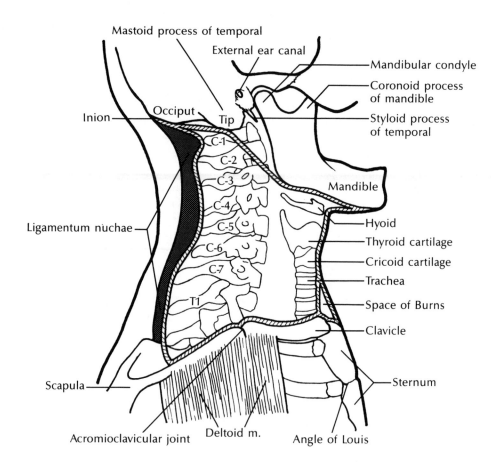

Illustration 2-8-A
Boundaries of the Superficial Fascia of the Neck

to form the apex of the triangle. The base of the triangle is formed by the middle third of the clavicle.

The omohyoid muscle (inferior belly) crosses the posterior triangle in a diagonal direction from above (anteriorly) to the angle of the base of the triangle (posteriorly) which is formed by the trapezius and the clavicle. The superficial fascia divides to envelop this muscle. Next, the layers of the fascia reunite between the muscle and the clavicle to form a ligament which helps to hold the muscle in place (ILLUSTRATION 2-9).

The superficial fascia also envelops the sternocleidomastoid and infrahyoid muscles (behind the sternocleidomastoid) as it completes its cylindrical formation around the neck. The anterior layer, as it envelops the infrahyoid muscles, attaches to the hyoid bone above and the sternum below. The lateral boundaries of the space of Burns (see above) are formed by the sternocleidomastoid (ILLUSTRATION 2-10). Within this space, we find the lower ends of the anterior jugular veins, a transverse connecting vein between the two and possibly a few lymph nodes.

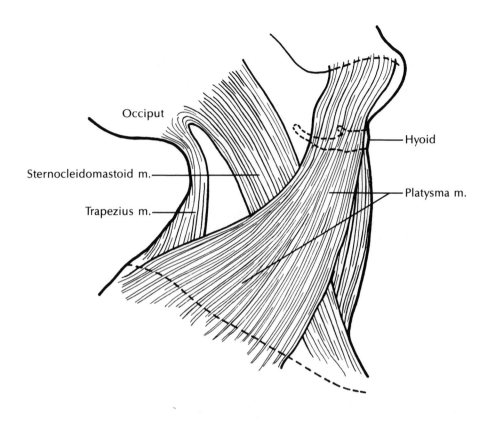

Illustration 2-8-B
Platysma Muscle

G. Overview

To summarize, we can view these fasciae of the neck as tubes within tubes (with the exception of the carotid sheaths) from the outside to the center. The superficial fascia is the outermost tube. It envelops the trapezius, inferior belly of the omohyoid, SCM and infrahyoid muscles.

The carotid sheaths (the only paired fascial tubes in the neck) are located antero-laterally to the vertebral column. They are divided into three longitudinally oriented compartments containing the carotid arteries (common carotid up to the bifurcation, then internal carotid above the bifurcation), internal jugular veins and vagus nerves.

The pretracheal fascia, lying anterior to the trachea and esophagus, connects the two carotid sheaths across the midline and helps envelop the thyroid gland. It contributes the anterior wall and inner lining of a fascial tube which contains the viscera as they pass through the neck; the carotid sheaths and prevertebral fascia also contribute to this tube (ILLUSTRATION 2-11).

The prevertebral fascia forms a cylinder enclosing the vertebral column and its related musculature. In front, it is divided into two lamina of which the anterior (alar lamina) contributes to the visceral tube illustrated above. Between these two lamina is a space which extends from the base of the skull into the upper thorax. This space

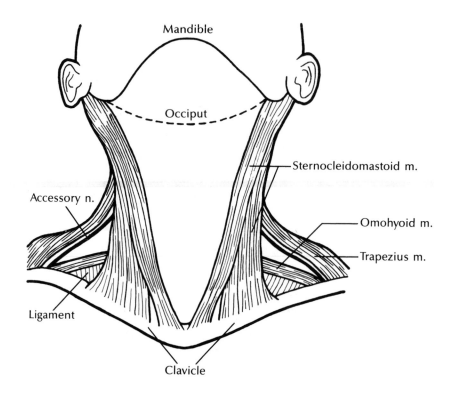

Illustration 2-9
Anterior View of Posterior Triangles of the Neck

is of interest to surgeons as a pathway for infection between the neck and the thorax, and to craniosacral therapists more because it offers some freedom of motion between the vertebral column and the cervical viscera.

The dura mater forms the watertight boundary of the semiclosed hydraulic system which we call the craniosacral system. The arachnoid is the meningeal layer with the greatest propensity to swell up with injury and/or toxicity, and can develop adhesions to the dura, both significant clinical problems. Adhesion of the arachnoid to the dura can cause a great deal of pain, not easily relieved by analgesics, acupuncture and the like. Craniosacral therapy will frequently help those suffering from this condition, but the pain often gets worse before it gets better.

III. HYOID BONE

A. Introduction

The hyoid bone, located in the anterior upper neck, is a beautifully designed mobile mooring station. Without it we would have no throat profile; our skin would go directly from mandible to sternum. Temporomandibular joint specialists often use X-ray studies

FRONT
OF NECK

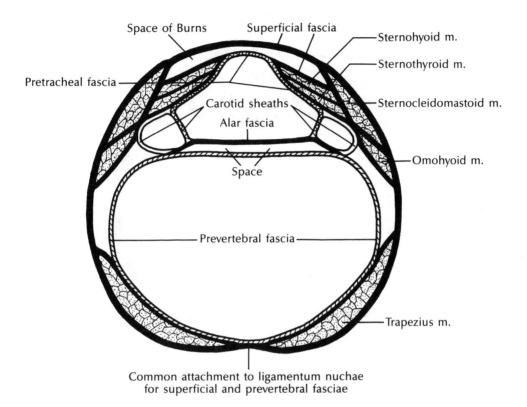

Illustration 2-10
Cross Section of Lower Neck
Showing Fascial Compartments

of the vertical level of the hyoid bone both diagnostically and as a prognostic indicator. Competent craniosacral therapy requires a detailed knowledge of this bone and its related anatomy.

B. Structure

The hyoid is an unpaired, U-shaped bone; the closed curve of the "U" is anterior and the arms are aimed posteriorly. The tips of the arms are suspended from the styloid processes of the temporal bones by the stylohyoid ligaments. Just as the mandible is a single bone joined to the temporal bones by the temporomandibular joints, so the hyoid bone may be thought of as a smaller version of the mandible, oriented in the same direction, and also joined to the temporal. The hyoid has five parts: the (unpaired) body, two greater cornua and two lesser cornua.

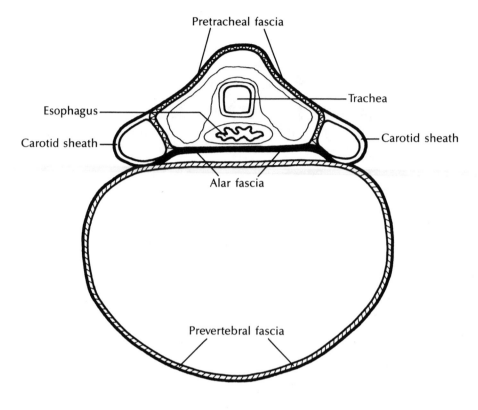

Illustration 2-11
Visceral Fascial Tube

The body of the hyoid is somewhat quadrilateral in shape and convex anteriorly. It is about 5cm across and 2.5cm or less in its vertical dimension; the widest dimension is across the neck on a horizontal plane. Its anterior surface is marked by a transverse ridge, and often by a vertical median ridge which divides it into lateral halves. The posterior surface is smooth, concave and directed a little bit downward or caudally. This surface is separated from the epiglottis by the thyrohyoid membrane and some loose connective tissue. The superior border of the body is somewhat rounded with the convexity up; the inferior border demonstrates an inferior concavity.

The greater cornua project posteriorly from the lateral body, forming the projections which give the hyoid its U-shape. They are about 3cm long, becoming more slender posteriorly. Each has a tubercle at the end.

The lesser cornua are small cone-shaped projections (slightly over 1cm long) which look like extensions of the transverse ridge of the body. They are roughly 6mm in diameter at the base and project from the body in a posterior and slightly superior direction. They are usually attached to the body by fibrous tissue, just above the greater cornua. Sometimes there is a rudimentary synovial joint between the lesser and greater cornua (ILLUSTRATION 2-12).

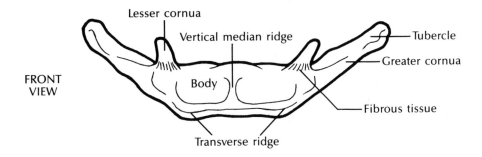

FRONT VIEW

Lesser cornua

Vertical median ridge

Tubercle

Greater cornua

Body

Fibrous tissue

Transverse ridge

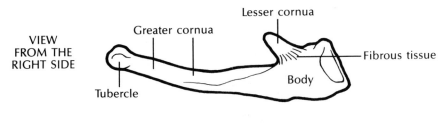

VIEW FROM THE RIGHT SIDE

Greater cornua

Lesser cornua

Fibrous tissue

Tubercle

Body

Illustration 2-12
Hyoid Bone

C. Hyoid attachments

There are 14 pair of muscles and connective tissue structures attaching to the hyoid, which is a considerable number for a bone this small. As we discuss these numerous attachments, keep in mind the functions of the hyoid: it participates in the movements of swallowing, talking, blowing a wind instrument and many other similar activities.

1. Muscles. The geniohyoid muscle inserts broadly on the front surface of the body of the hyoid, above and below the transverse ridge. It originates from the mental spine on the internal surface of the mandible. Contraction of the muscle elevates the hyoid (when the hyoid is not fixed from below), or helps lower the mandible (when the hyoid is fixed). Innervation is from C1, whose fibers hitch a ride with the hypoglossal nerves in order to reach their destination (CHAPTER 1, SECTION X).

The hyoglossus muscle arises from the lateral hyoid body and the upper surface of the greater cornua. It ascends into the tongue and aids in tongue movement.

The mylohyoid is an almost transversely oriented muscle which arises from the circumference of the internal surface of the mandible, and inserts into a median raphe (extending from the hyoid to the mandible) and the anterior body of the hyoid. It forms the floor of the mouth. Its contraction raises the hyoid.

The sternohyoid is a thin strap muscle arising from the medial ends of the clavicles, the back of the manubrium and the sternoclavicular ligaments. It inserts on the inferior body of the hyoid. At their origin, the two halves are separated by 2.5cm or more; as they ascend they converge so that their medial borders come in contact about

3-4cm below the insertion. Contraction of this muscle lowers the hyoid during swallowing. Innervation is from fibers of segments C1 through C3, via the ansa cervicalis nerve.

The omohyoid muscle is divided into two bellies by a central tendon. The inferior belly arises from the upper scapula, extends forward to the clavicle (where it attaches by a fibrous band) and then runs deep to the sternocleidomastoid muscle and inserts on its own central tendon (which is held in place by a specialized process of its investing fascia that attaches to the clavicle and first rib). The superior belly ascends close to the lateral border of the sternohyoid muscle and inserts into the lower border of the hyoid body lateral to the sternohyoid insertion. Contraction of the omohyoid lowers the hyoid. Innervation is the same as that of the sternohyoid (ILLUSTRATIONS 2-13-A and 2-13-B).

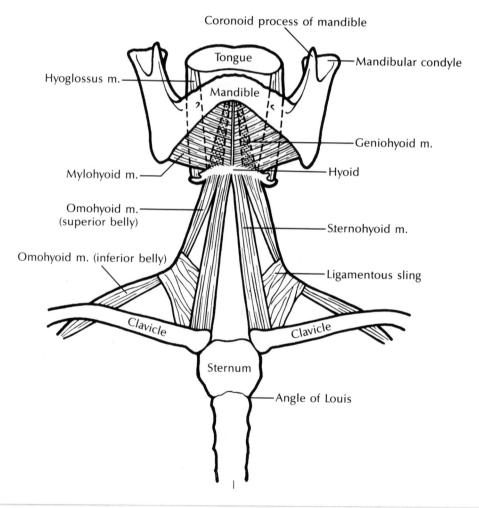

Illustration 2-13-A
Anterior View of Muscular Attachments to the Hyoid

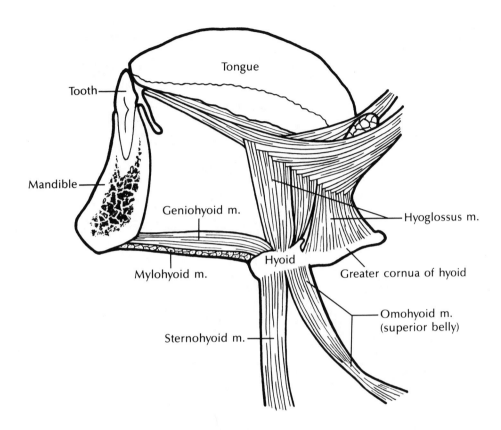

Illustration 2-13-B
Lateral View of Muscular Attachments to the Hyoid

2. Other attachments. The thyrohyoid membrane is broad and fibroelastic. It originates from the lateral border of the hyoid body, passes behind the hyoid and attaches to the upper border of the thyroid cartilage (and, in passing, the inferior dorsal edge of the hyoid body and the greater cornua). There is a bursa between the membrane and the hyoid which facilitates movement during the swallowing process. There is a thickened area in the middle of the membrane, known as the thyrohyoid ligament. The lateral regions of the membrane are thinner, and are pierced by the superior laryngeal vessels and the internal branches of the superior laryngeal nerve. The anterior surface of the membrane is covered by the infrahyoid muscles and the hyoid body.

The hyoepiglottic ligament connects the hyoid body to the epiglottis.

The thyrohyoid muscle (a continuation of the sternothyroid muscle) arises either from the inferior hyoid body or, more commonly, the inferior border of the greater cornua (ILLUSTRATION 2-14). It acts to shorten the distance between the thyroid cartilage and the hyoid bone; its effect depends upon which of these structures is fixed. It is innervated by the 1st cervical nerve segment traveling with the hypoglossal nerve.

When present, the levator glandulae thyroideae muscle attaches the isthmus of the thyroid gland to the inferior border of the hyoid body. Its contraction raises the isthmus toward the hyoid bone, the purpose of which is unclear.

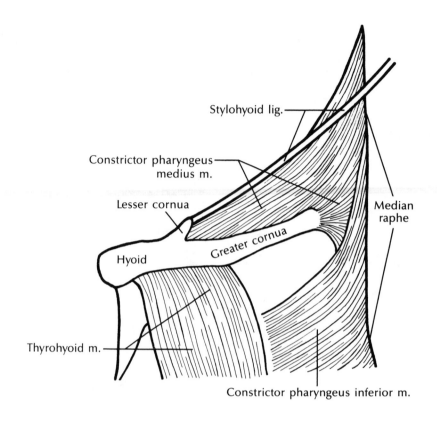

Illustration 2-14
Thyrohyoid and Constrictor Pharyngeus
Medius Muscles

The lateral thyrohyoid ligaments are round, elastic, cordlike structures (actually the lateral boundaries of the thyrohyoid membrane) arising from the tubercles of the greater cornua. They connect the greater cornua to the superior cornua of the thyroid cartilage.

The constrictor pharyngis medius muscle arises from the length of the greater cornua, the lesser cornua and the stylohyoid ligament (SECTION III.B). The fibers fan out from their origin and insert into the posterior median raphe. Contraction of this muscle holds the hyoid bone in a posterior position. Its action is coordinated with those of other muscles during the swallowing process (ILLUSTRATION 2-14).

The digastric and stylohyoid muscles insert on the greater cornua near their junctions with the hyoid body. It is actually the ligamentous loops on each side (through which the tendons of the digastric muscles pass) that attach to the hyoid bone. The stylohyoid arises from the temporal styloid processes and acts to retract the hyoid bone in a posterior direction. It also has a significant effect on temporal bone function (ILLUSTRATION 2-15). Innervation is by the facial nerve. The digastric muscle will be described in chapter 3, section III.E.5.a.

The stylohyoid ligaments connect the lesser cornua to the temporal styloid processes, providing the conduction pathway by which the infrahyoid muscles influence temporal bone function in the craniosacral sense.

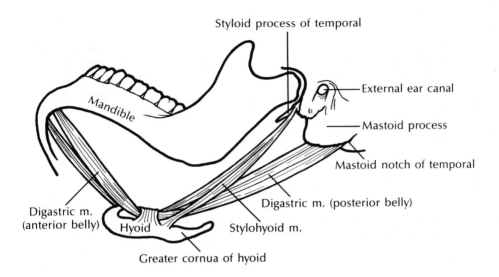

Illustration 2-15
Digastric and Stylohyoid Muscles

The chondroglossus muscles arise medially to the bases of the lesser cornua. These muscles ascend about 2.5cm to the tongue and blend with its intrinsic muscles.

D. Functional muscle groupings

1. Muscles which depress the hyoid. These are the infrahyoid muscles (sternohyoid, omohyoid and thyrohyoid) discussed in section III.C.1. They also act to fix the hyoid in place. The thyrohyoid is actually a continuation of the sternothyroid muscle which runs from the sternum to the thyroid cartilage.

2. Muscles which elevate the hyoid. These are the geniohyoid, mylohyoid and digastric. They depend upon a stabilized mandible for their actions, i.e., hyoid elevation is dependent (via the mandible) upon the masseters, the medial pterygoids and the temporalis muscles. Coordinated function in this situation requires integration of the trigeminal system (which supplies the muscles of mastication) with those nerves supplying the hyoid muscles (i.e., trigeminal, facial and hypoglossal). The hypoglossal is a conductor of fibers from C1 only; its central nucleus is not directly involved in motor innervation to these muscles.

The muscles which elevate the hyoid bone when the mandible is fixed will help lower the mandible (open the mouth) when the hyoid is fixed (stabilized) from below by the infrahyoid muscles.

3. Muscles which retract the hyoid. These are the constrictor pharyngis medius and stylohyoid muscles. Without them, the hyoid would tend to displace forward. The stylohyoid, as noted above, connects the hyoid to the temporal bone, with important craniosacral system implications.

I was first exposed to the effects of hyoid bone problems in the craniosacral system in a very personal way. Subsequent to a rather severe throat infection, my own hyoid began to feel as though it was being pulled in many directions at once. The discomfort was quite palpable between the hyoid and the thyroid cartilage on the right side. Oddly enough, I also began to notice that as I wrote I was reversing letters, as a dyslexic would tend to do. I could see the reversal with my eyes, but my hand wrote the words incorrectly even as I watched. It was a rather strange experience. Fortunately, my friend Dr. Richard MacDonald came to town while I was suffering this problem. He applied craniosacral therapy and discovered that my right temporal bone was almost totally immobilized. His impression was that the stylohyoideus muscle on the right was in a hypertonic state and interfering with temporal bone motion. He successfully released the hyoid and its related muscles, including the right stylohyoid. I am pleased to say that my right temporal bone is again functional, my energy level is improved and my handwriting, although still difficult to read, is no longer subject to letter reversal. My experience has shown that many problems related to dyslexia are etiologically related to right temporal bone dysfunction (UPLEDGER 1983:261).

E. Overview

The hyoid is continually adjusted in its position by three groups of muscles: those muscles which depress it or fix it from below; those which retract it or fix it posteriorly; and those which elevate it or fix it from above.

The hyoid offers grounding for the hyoglossus, genioglossus and chondroglossus muscles to the tongue; controlled tongue movement is important in a variety of our everyday activities. A lack of positional control of the hyoid bone may show itself as a tongue dysfunction (in speech, swallowing, etc.).

Many muscles which seem unrelated to the hyoid can influence its function via the fasciae and ligaments discussed above. The thyrohyoid membrane connects the hyoid to the thyroid cartilage, and forms the middle and lateral thyrohyoid ligaments. The bursa between this membrane and the posterior surface of the body of the hyoid facilitates hyoid movement.

The hyoid is attached to the prevertebral and superficial fasciae discussed above in sections II.C and II.F; abnormal tension in these fasciae can cause hyoid dysfunction. The stylohyoid ligaments connect the hyoid to the temporal bones. These three bones, plus the occipital base, form a circle through which all food and air must pass in order to enter the body.

I have seen many post upper respiratory infection and "flu" cases wherein a lingering cough persisted for weeks or even months. I have just completed the case of a 76-year-old woman who suffered from a chronic cough "deep in the throat" for almost a year following a bout with bronchitis. She had been treated by her family doctor with antibiotics, expectorants and subsequently with cough suppressants. Her cough continued, and she complained of "thick mucus" in her throat all the time. Release of the hyoid, its related soft tissues, the temporals and the occiput ended the cough syndrome in one treatment session.

Since most of the hyoid muscles are supplied by cranial nerves (V, VII and XII) and the upper cervical segments (C1, 2 and 3), the craniosacral system must be in good working order to insure proper function of the hyoid. Release of the occipital cranial base is imperative, as is functional balancing of the cervical spine. This mandates that special attention be paid to the cervico-thoracic junction through release of the thoracic inlet.

IV. CARTILAGES OF THE LARYNX

A. Thyroid cartilage

The air passage in the neck must remain open at all times. It is therefore surrounded by cartilages which prevent its collapse. The thyroid cartilage is the largest of these cartilages. It contributes the anterior and lateral walls of the larynx, an organ of the respiratory system. During fetal development, this cartilage is formed in two bilateral parts, which join at the midline as development continues to form a rather acute angle. This angle is what you feel as the protuberance ("Adam's apple") in the front of your throat. If you palpate carefully on the midline, you can feel a notch (the superior thyroid notch) on the antero-superior thyroid cartilage. As the two halves of the thyroid cartilage extend laterally, they curve somewhat to form a semi-rounded anterior wall for the throat. At the lateral borders there are projections (superior and inferior cornua) extending vertically upward and downward. The structure of the thyroid cartilage can be compared to an old fashioned canvas litter or stretcher. The cornua represent the handles and the anteriorly placed rounded cartilage represents the canvas carrier part (ILLUSTRATION 2-16).

B. Cricoid cartilage

The upper border of the thyroid cartilage is continuous with the hyoid via the thyrohyoid membrane described in section III.C.2. The thyroid cartilage's inferior cornua are continuous (via articular surfaces) with the posterior lateral surfaces of the cricoid cartilage below. The cricoid cartilage forms the lower part of the laryngeal wall and the entry into the trachea. It is thicker and stronger than the thyroid cartilage, and is the only cartilage structure forming a complete ring around the larynx or trachea. The cricoid cartilage is about 0.6cm high anteriorly and 3cm high posteriorly. This height differential allows for forward bending of the neck without compressing the anterior cartilages.

Most tracheostomies (surgical openings directly into the trachea) are done just inferior to the lower margin of the cricoid cartilage, and above the uppermost tracheal ring.

A thick ligament on the anterior midline connects the cricoid cartilage with the thyroid cartilage. In addition, the entire upper border anterior to the cricothyroid articulations offers attachment to a broad cricothyroid membrane, which runs upward behind the thyroid cartilage to form the conus elasticus. This structure attaches to the inner surface of the thyroid cartilage and to the arytenoid cartilages which are discussed below, and forms the vocal ligaments which underlie the vocal cords.

The vocal cords are connective tissues specialized for sound production. They attach to the thyroid cartilage anteriorly at the midline and are here immovable. The

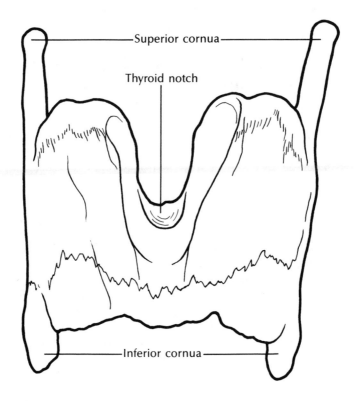

Illustration 2-16
Anterior View of Thyroid Cartilage

posterior attachments are to the arytenoid cartilages which move transverely in and out, allowing the posterior ends of the vocal cords to move together and apart as you sing or speak. The vocal cords thus form the two legs of an isosceles triangle which has its apex at the internal surface of the thyroid cartilage. The base of the triangle, of variable length, is determined by the distance between the movable arytenoid cartilages.

C. Other cartilages

The paired arytenoid cartilages are found at the upper dorsal aspect of the cricoid cartilage. They are somewhat pyramidal in shape. The dorsal surfaces are triangular and give attachment to the transverse and oblique arytenoid muscles which connect the two cartilages. These muscles assist in controlling the distance between the arytenoid cartilages and thus the vocal cords.

The antero-lateral surfaces of the arytenoid cartilages give attachment to the vestibular ligaments, and to the thyroarytenoid and vocalis muscles (which act on the vocal cords during speech). These surfaces also have numerous mucous glands. The medial triangular surfaces, also called the laryngeal surfaces, are covered by mucous membranes.

The bases of the arytenoid "pyramids" project laterally and give attachment to the cricoarytenoid muscles and, more anteriorly, to the vocal ligaments. They also provide the joint surfaces for the cricoarytenoid joints, which allow sliding between the cartilages which open or narrow the airway.

The corniculate cartilages, two small cartilages which sit atop the apices of the arytenoid cartilages, are considered vestigial in humans. Earlier in mammalian evolution they probably helped to close the esophagus during swallowing in order to prevent regurgitation.

The cuneiform cartilages, about 1.3cm long, are very thin and curved. They are located in the aryepiglottic folds, just in front of the arytenoid cartilages. They are probably also vestigial.

The epiglottis is an unpaired, thin, leaf-shaped, yellow elastic cartilage. It projects upward toward the root of the tongue from its anchor on the posterior surface of the hyoid. Its connection to the hyoid is by the hyoepiglottic ligament; it is also attached to the thyroid cartilage by the thyroepiglottic ligament. The free borders of the epiglottis are covered by mucous membrane. The aryepiglottic folds are attached to it at its lateral edges, near its root attachment. The epiglottis moves up to open (during breathing) and down and posterior to close (during swallowing) the airway.

V. SUPPORTING STRUCTURES AND FUNCTION OF THE LARYNX

The larynx is the organ which enables us to communicate vocally. It is located in the neck at the levels of vertebrae C4 through C6, and connects the pharynx to the trachea. It opens and closes the airway through the functioning of the epiglottis. Aspiration of food or drink into the respiratory passageways is due to failure of the epiglottis to close. This section will examine some of the supporting structures of the larynx.

A. Ligaments

Extrinsic ligaments are those which connect the larynx to outside structures. Intrinsic ligaments interconnect laryngeal structures. The same terminology will be applied to muscles.

Extrinsic ligaments of the larynx include the two lateral thyrohyoid ligaments (SECTION III.C.2), middle thyrohyoid ligament (SECTION III.C.2) and broad thyrohyoid membrane which connect the thyroid cartilage and hyoid; and the hyoepiglottic ligament, an unpaired elastic band which connects the anterior surface of the epiglottis to the upper aspect of the hyoid.

The (intrinsic) cricotracheal ligament is a fibrous membranous structure which connects the cricoid cartilage with the upper tracheal cartilage ring.

B. Muscles

The muscles acting on the hyoid were described in section III.D. There are only two extrinsic muscles inserting on the larynx, the sternothyroid and thyrohyoid. The sternothyroid connects the sternum to the thyroid cartilage. It originates from the posterior surface of the manubrium inferior to the sternohyoid muscle, and from the cartilage of the first, and sometimes the second, rib. It lies deep to the sternohyoid muscle. When the sternothyroid contracts, it pulls the thyroid cartilage and thus the whole larynx inferiorly. Innervation is from the upper three cervical segments via the ansa cervicalis nerve.

The small, quadrangular thyrohyoid muscles arise from the oblique line of the thyroid cartilage and insert into the inferior border of the greater cornua of the hyoid. They are, for all practical purposes, continuations of the sternothyroid muscles. Contraction of the thyrohyoids shortens the distance beween the thyroid cartilage and the hyoid bone. If the hyoid is fixed, they raise the thyroid cartilage. If the thyroid cartilage is fixed from below, they will pull the hyoid bone inferiorly. Innervation is by fibers of C1 traveling with the hypoglossal nerve.

C. External spatial relationships

The larynx glides up and down as you swallow. Obstructions to this freedom of movement are felt as unpleasant sensations and difficulty in swallowing. It only takes a tiny adhesion to create a large subjective sense of restriction.

Laterally and anteriorly, the thyroid gland is in contact with the thyroid and cricoid cartilages; the thyroid gland isthmus is either just below or directly in front of the cricoid cartilage. The gland's upper poles extend up over the thyroid cartilage bilaterally. There is an adherent zone of the inner surface of the thyroid gland which attaches either to the lateral cricoid cartilage or to the tracheal ring just below the cartilage.

The thyroid and cricoid cartilages are largely covered anteriorly by the infrahyoid muscles (SECTION III.D). There is little between the larynx and the skin of the anterior neck besides these muscles, their fasciae and the superficial fascia (SECTION II.F). Posterolaterally, the larynx is adjacent but not adherent to the carotid sheaths. The larynx is separated posteriorly from the trachea by a space between its fascia and the pretracheal fascia, allowing for independent movement between the two organs.

The vagus nerve, as it passes downward through the neck within the carotid sheathes, gives off the superior laryngeal nerves (each of which divides into internal and external branches) and recurrent laryngeal nerves. These nerves are all closely related to the trachea, esophagus and the larynx. The recurrent laryngeal nerve (along with accompanying inferior thyroid vessel branches) enters the larynx just behind the cricothyroid joints on either side of the larynx. The superior laryngeal nerves are just medial to the internal and external carotid arteries as they descend before branching. The internal branch of the superior laryngeal nerve (along with associated vessels which branch off of thyroid vessels) passes over the lateral thyrohyoid ligament before entering the larynx; the external branch accompanies the inferior laryngeal constrictor muscles which attach to the thyroid cartilage. The nerve branches will frequently supply the constrictor muscle, then travel on to supply the cricothyroid muscles which are so important in vocalization.

D. Internal structure

The internal cavity of the larynx extends downward from its superior opening or entrance. This entrace is bounded by many structures. The most important are the epiglottis, the apices of the arytenoid cartilages, the corniculate cartilages, the interarytenoid notch and the folds of mucous membrane on either side. These membrane folds (called the aryepiglottic folds [see SECTION IV.C]) enclose the muscles and ligaments which connect the sides of the epiglottis to the apices of the arytenoid cartilages; the posterior margins are connected to the cuneiform cartilages. The inferior opening or exit of the larynx (into the trachea) is the lower border of the cricoid cartilage ring.

Inside the larynx are the intrinsic muscles and ligaments which enable us to perform many crucial functions, including swallowing, talking and singing. The intrinsic ligaments include the elastic membrane which extends from the entrance to the exit at the cricoid cartilage. Below the vocal cords, this membrane is called the conus elasticus, or cricothyroid membrane. Above the vocal cords it is simply known as the cranial portion of the elastic membrane of the larynx. The conus elasticus connects the thyroid cartilage to the cricoid and arytenoid cartilages. Laterally, it is covered by the cricothyroid muscles and the anastomotic junction of the two cricothyroid arteries which pass through it.

There are many other intrinsic ligaments of the larynx. The most important among them include the articular capsules which enclose the articulations between the inferior cornua of the thyroid cartilage and the cricoid cartilage; cricoarytenoid capsules and ligaments which connect the arytenoid cartilages to the cricoid cartilage; and the thyroepiglottic ligament, which connects the epiglottis to the thyroid cartilage. This last is a midline unpaired ligament which attaches to the internal surface of the thyroid cartilage just below the superior thyroid notch. Its main function is to allow relatively free movement of the two structures.

The actual cavity in the larynx is usually divided into two subcavities by anatomists. The projections of the vocal folds and vocal cords are used as a boundary. The part of the cavity above the vocal folds/cords is known as the vestibule. The portion below is called the ventricle.

The intrinsic muscles of the larynx function in vocalization. They are called the cricothyroids, posterior cricoarytenoids, lateral cricoarytenoids, arytenoids and thyroarytenoids. These muscles in concert control the vocal cords, and thus speech and singing, via the arytenoid cartilages.

The intralaryngeal blood vessels (arteries and veins) are derived from the superior and inferior thyroid vessels. Thus, the arteries are subbranches originally derived from the carotid arteries, and the veins eventually empty into the internal jugular veins. The lymphatic vessels of the larynx are largely responsible for problems such as hoarseness and loss of voice when their function is impaired. These lymphatics drain either into lymph nodes located near the bifurcations of the common carotid arteries or into nodes in the tracheal or deep cervical area. It is important to note that innervation to the intrinsic muscles of the larynx is from the vagus system. The vessels and lymph nodes are supplied by sympathetic nerve fibers.

VI. SPACES OF THE NECK

A. Below the hyoid

Most important in the application of craniosacral therapy to the neck is an appreciation of the spaces between fasciae and structures which allow freedom and independent movement. Below the hyoid bone, the interfascial spaces are known as the pretracheal space, the retrovisceral space, the visceral space, the potential space within the carotid sheath and the space between the two lamina of the prevertebral fascia.

1. The **pretracheal space** (which encloses the thyroid gland) is bounded above by the attachment of the infrahyoid muscles and fasciae to the hyoid bone and the thyroid cartilage, below by the junction of the fibrous pericardium with the sternum (at the level of vertebra T4, at the aortic arch), anteriorly by the fascia of the larynx and posteriorly by the fascia of the trachea.

2. The **retrovisceral space** has two divisions. Superiorly, it is called the retropharyngeal space, and has the skull as its upper limit behind the pharynx. As the pharynx extends downward and is continuous with the esophagus, the retropharyngeal space continues downward as the retroesophageal space.

The retrovisceral space is bounded below by the fusion of connective tissue/fasciae on the posterior surface of the esophagus to the prevertebral fascia (SECTION II.C); this fusion occurs in the upper mediastinum. Thus, the space lies between the posterior walls of the pharynx-esophagus complex and the vertebral column, and allows independent motion between these two structures.

The "visceral space" is a term applied to the potential space between the viscera of the neck and their investing fasciae. Since these fasciae are rather tightly adhered to the viscera, the "space" is of little or no significance in craniosacral therapeutic techniques aimed at the establishment of free and easy mobilization of the structures of the neck.

3. Carotid space. Another instance of potential space, perhaps more significant to our purpose, is that within the carotid sheath on both sides of the neck. Many pathologists believe that infection is able to spread downward within this sheath into the mediastinum; this view is still somewhat controversial. I do believe that an awareness of this potential space is helpful both diagnostically and therapeutically to the craniosacral therapist. When fibrosis, adhesions, edema, etc., occur within the carotid sheath, the effect upon blood flow in and out of the skull, and upon vagus nerve function, can become significant (if not devastating) clinically. Infection and other problems within this sheath may arise from the lymph nodes within the sheath and/or from internal jugular vein thrombosis. Therapeutic intent focused upon this area with cooperative imaging between client and therapist can be quite effective.

The most graphic example I have seen of this type of situation is that of a 38-year-old woman accused of having many neurotic symptoms related to headache, fatigue, lack of enthusiasm and depression. Previously, she had undergone a carotid angiogram in which radio-opaque dye was injected into the carotid artery in order to visualize the blood flow to the brain. The whole craniosacral system was inhibited on that side of the head. After releasing the cervical fasciae in the region of the carotid sheath, the "neurotic" symptoms have improved slowly but consistently and the craniosacral system is functioning much more smoothly.

I have another case which appears to be related to problems with the carotid sheath. This patient has been suffering from "migraine headache" for many years. At age 63, a neurosurgeon decided to operate and remove a portion of the sympathetic nerve plexus from the left carotid artery in order to stop the pain. The operation was a failure in terms of symptom relief. Palpation indicated that the left carotid sheath was essentially immobile. To date I have been unsuccessful in mobilizing the sheath. The headaches are somewhat better controlled with regular craniosacal therapy, but the cranial dysfunctions related to the carotid sheath persist. So far, any help has been palliative and temporary. I have seen this woman (now 65 years of age) on a weekly basis for almost 20 visits. We'll keep trying, but the post-operative adhesions are proving most difficult to overcome.

No matter the source, chronic and ongoing symptoms related to obstructions and restrictions within the confines of the carotid sheath can be a most puzzling and frustrating problem to patients and physicians alike. It is the kind of problem which will often be referred inappropriately for psychiatric help. You should recall that the carotid sheaths (SECTION II.E) have their upper attachment to the base of the skull. Via these attachments, they can adversely influence craniosacral system function; they can, conversely, be favorably influenced by craniosacral therapeutic techniques aimed at mobilization of the temporo-occipito-sphenoidal contributions to the floor of the cranial vault. The V-spread technique can be applied through the carotid sheaths.

4. "Pre-prevertebral" space. Another infrahyoid space in the neck is found between the two layers of the anterior expanse of the prevertebral fascia as it travels around the front of the vertebral bodies. This space encloses the muscles acting on the vertebral column as well as their ancillary blood vessels and nerves. Between the attachments of the prevertebral fascia to the transverse processes of the vertebrae, the anterior expanse of fascia is separated into two lamina which are able to move independently of each other (SECTION II.C). The anterior (alar) lamina forms the posterior boundary of the retrovisceral space, and is thus interposed between the retrovisceral space and the posterior (prevertebral) lamina. One might therefore call the space between the two lamina the "pre-prevertebral space" (the term prevertebral space would then be reserved for the space between the posterior lamina and vertebral column). This space actually extends from the base of the skull well into the thorax, often as low as the respiratory diaphragm.

Thus, we have the retrovisceral space, pre-prevertebral space and prevertebral space, all between the vertebrae and the viscera of the neck. Natural selection has obviously dictated that we have the ability to move the vertebral column independently from the cervical viscera.

B. Above the hyoid

1. Introduction. Above the hyoid there are fewer fasciae, but more spaces. The craniosacral therapist needs a working knowledge of this area, which relates to the cranium, palate, mandible and its joints and the rest of the face.

There are three suprahyoid fasciae: superficial fascia, prevertebral fascia and buc-copharyngeal fascia. The spaces bounded by them may likewise be divided into three categories. First are the intrafascial spaces which are formed to accommodate a structure. These spaces have no open communication with any other space. They are formed by splitting a fascia into two lamina to form a completely closed pouch. Second are the intercommunicating spaces, found principally around the pharynx. These spaces are located between the pharyngeal wall and the fascial layers. Third are the blind spaces which are usually not "open." They are potential spaces, i.e., between two layers of fascia which can be separated by very little pressure (as from fluid) to form a blind pouch. Some of these pouches are located within the pharyngeal wall deep to the buc-copharyngeal fascia.

2. Intrafascial spaces. The "pre-prevertebral space" discussed in section VI.A.4 begins at the base of the skull, and can therefore be included in this category. All of the remaining suprahyoid intrafascial spaces are formed by a splitting of the superficial layer of upper cervical fascia as it attaches to the bones of the head and face. Recall that these spaces are all closed. Infections of any of these spaces or their contents can only spread by means of rupture through one of their fascial walls.

a. Submaxillary gland spaces. These spaces are often called submandibular or, less often, sublingual or submental. This variable terminology can obviously be a source of confusion. The superficial fascia in the region between the hyoid bone and the mandible on the underside of the chin simply splits into two lamina in order to accommodate the submaxillary glands (which secrete saliva into the oral cavity) and their associated lymph nodes. The external layer of the capsule formed is very strong. The thinner internal layer is perforated by the duct of the gland and its associated vessels and nerves. The gland is not freely movable; there is a lot of connective tissue which penetrates the gland and binds it to the capsule.

Some anatomists refer to the space between the superficial fascia of the suprahyoid region and the mylohyoid muscle as the submaxillary or submandibular space. This usage adds further confusion. This space does exist but is certainly not an intrafascial space. It is a space between two separate layers of fascia.

b. Parotid gland spaces. These enclose the parotid (salivary) glands and associated lymph nodes, the facial nerve and its communications with the great auricular and auriculotemporal nerves and the external carotid artery (which branches within the capsule of the gland). The common facial vein unites with the auricular vein within the gland to form the external jugular vein, which passes through the parotid gland space on each side. The duct of the gland passes through the internal fascia of the capsule. The lymph glands associated with the parotid gland and its space drain into the superficial and deep cervical channels. Like the submaxillary gland, the parotid gland is well attached by fibrous tissue (which completely penetrates the gland) to the walls of its capsule.

The superficial fascia which forms the parotid gland spaces is attached above to the bones of the zygomatic arch and below to the mandible. The parotid gland space is completely above the mandible. The stylohyoid ligament partially separates the parotid from the submaxillary glands.

c. Masticator spaces. These are formed as the superficial cervical fascia on each side of the neck splits into two lamina (external and internal) above the inferior border of the ramus (at the angle) of the mandible. The space formed by this division accommodates the ramus as it goes up to the temporomandibular joint, as well as the masseter, medial pterygoid and lower temporalis muscles. The space is bounded posteriorly (behind the ramus) by fusion of the two lamina; anteriorly by fascial attachment to the anterior border of the ramus, to the maxilla and to the temporalis insertion onto the mandible; and superiorly by the attachment of the fascia to the skull on the deep side of the temporalis muscle and to the temporal fascia superficially.

There is some extension of the masticator space into the deep anterior pterygopalatine fossa. It accommodates all of the nerves and vessels which service the masticatory system, and contains much loose connective tissue and fat. Its anatomy will be further discussed in chapter 3.

d. Mandibular spaces. These are formed by the superficial cervical fascia as it comes forward and a little upward from the hyoid to the mandible. The fascia splits into two lamina to accommodate the body of the mandible. The mandibular "space" thus formed is actually a potential space, i.e., where the fascia is easily separated from the bone. The outer lamina attaches to the lower border of the external mandible. The inner lamina covers the internal surface of the bone up to the attachment of the mylohyoid muscle (about 2cm above the inferior border of the bone). The mandibular space is bounded antero-medially by the attachment of the digastric muscle; postero-laterally by the attachments of the medial pterygoids; anteriorly by the attachments of the fasciae; and postero-inferiorly by fusion of the two lamina as they move away from the mandible.

e. Craniosacral considerations. These intrafascial spaces are significant to the craniosacral therapist because problems within the spaces can change the size of the space (distend it) so that the involved fascia becomes less mobile. Also, previous inflammation can make the fascia less pliable, thus interfering with good fascial function. You must determine whether there is active inflammation present, or whether the dysfunction results from previous inflammation which is no longer active but which may still require treatment. If the inflammation is active, it will feel warmer and radiate more palpable energy. If you determine that it is active, induce mobility more from the periphery of the space. Allow time for the body to do its work as you enhance the circulation of body fluids into the area from the adjacent tissues. Gradually work your way into the center. Do not attack the center of the actual inflamed fascial space; you may cause increased tissue resistance and therefore increased rigidity. This works against you. Chip away gently and subtly from around the edges. Use the V-spread or direction of energy technique, which enhances the body's healing process and therefore its ability to effectively destroy invading infectious organisms. Gradually, after you feel the rigidity relaxing, begin to induce ever-increasing movement to the involved fascial sheets.

3. Intercommunicating spaces.

a. Introduction. Intercommunicating spaces are located between the superficial cervical fascia and the visceral structures of the upper neck, and communicate freely around the muscles which they contain. They actually form a comparmentalized ring around the pharynx above the hyoid bone. These spaces are subject to infection from the intrafascial spaces and the mandible (externally) and the pharynx (internally). They receive lymphatic drainage from the nose, throat and jaw; when lymph node protection is overwhelmed by infection and the node breaks down, the spaces are vulnerable to abscess formation. The infection may then spread because the spaces intercommunicate with each other.

b. Retropharyngeal space. This is the intercommunicating space behind the pharynx and in front of the alar lamina of the prevertebral fascia. Its upper boundary is the base of the skull; below, it is continuous with the retrovisceral space (SECTION VI.A.2). It forms the posterior part of the visceral compartment of the neck, communicates with the pretracheal space, ends at the bifurcation of the trachea and is separated from the pre-prevertebral space by the alar fascia (SECTION VI.A.4). The communications of this space mean that infection can spread through the anterior and posterior mediastinum without having to perforate a fascial wall. The retropharyngeal space contains loose connective tissue and some fat cells, and enhances the ability of the vertebral column to move independently from the viscera of the neck. When we perform anterior and posterior fascial traction techniques on the neck, we test the mobility between the vertebral column, the cervical viscera, the fasciae and the spaces which separate them.

c. Lateral pharyngeal spaces. These are continuous with the retropharyngeal space, providing the lateral contributions of the circle of spaces around the pharynx. Actually, the lateral and retropharyngeal spaces may be thought of as a horseshoe-shaped space which wraps around the pharynx. The lateral spaces are filled with loose connective tissue. They are bounded laterally by the fasciae of the pterygoid muscles and the sheaths of the parotid glands; medially by the fasciae which cover the pharynx; superiorly by the base of the skull; inferiorly by fusion and attachment of the fascial lamina to the sheaths of the submaxillary glands, which blend (at the level of the hyoid) with the sheaths of the posterior belly of the digastric and stylohyoid muscles; and posteriorly by the carotid sheaths. These spaces are crossed by the styloglossus and stylopharyngeus muscles, and communicate with the spaces of the floor of the mouth. Infections from the teeth or from the tonsillar region of the pharynx may be transmitted to the lateral and thence to the retropharyngeal spaces.

d. Submandibular space. This space is also referred to as the submaxillary space (no doubt to increase your confusion). It provides the anterior portion of the spaces around the pharynx, communicating with the other spaces described above. It is bounded inferiorly by the superficial cervical fascia between the mandible and the hyoid bone; posteriorly by the hyoid; and superiorly by the mucous membrane of the mouth and the tongue. This space is subdivided by the mylohyoid muscle, fascia of the anterior digastric and by the genioglossus and geniohyoid muscles.

That part of the submandibular space above the mylohyoid muscles is often referred to as the sublingual space. It contains loose connective tissue and the sublingual glands, and is traversed by the hypoglossal and lingual nerves, as well as by the duct of the submandibular gland and a variable part of that gland.

e. Clinical significance. Infection can spread from a lower tooth into the sub-mandibular space and thence to the mediastinum via the communications with the lateral and retropharyngeal spaces. Mobilization of the fasciae and other structures which relate to these spaces enhances the drainage of toxic fluids, as well as circulation of fresh blood with its infection-fighting antibodies and blood cells to the areas involved. Thus, gentle craniosacral techniques applied to the neck provide an excellent therapeutic approach to problems ranging from infected teeth to tonsillitis, mastoiditis and any other "-itis" of the head and neck.

4. Blind pouches. The third category of suprahyoid spaces are the "blind pouches." Many of these are actually potential spaces which are easily created by pressure from fluid, pus, etc. For example, the pharyngeal constrictor muscles are covered by buccopharyngeal fascia. The attachment is loose, and a potential space exists between the muscle and the fascia. External force (usually fluid pressure) can form a blind pouch which can, if further pressured, rupture into the lateral and/or retropharyngeal spaces.

The tonsils are loosely connected to the walls of the pharynx. Infection of the tonsils can create blind pouches as it separates (through pressure) the mucous membrane from the underlying tissues of the wall. These blind pouches are sometimes extended to the hard palate and/or to the opening of the auditory tube into the pharynx. They may also extend downward into the peripharyngeal spaces described in section VI.B.3, thus gaining eventual access to the mediastinum.

In this situation, gentle tissue mobilization is again the therapy of choice. Infection often impairs the host's immunological resistance. Craniosacral techniques aimed at the reinforcement of physiological motion assist the body's inherent resistance to pathogens.

VII. ANATOMY OF THE NECK: SUMMARY

In this chapter we have considered in a rather detailed manner the functional anatomy of the neck from a clinical point of view, and more specifically from a craniosacral therapist's point of view. We have seen how the fascial planes and compartments serve to separate and to provide mobility within the neck for the vital structures which pass through it. Vulnerabilities and routes of entry for treating hands have been noted. It is my hope that the neck now seems more accessible to you.

3.

TEMPOROMANDIBULAR JOINT

CHAPTER 3

I. INTRODUCTION

A Buddhist teaching says that the only thing upon which we may rely is change. That is, the conditions which prevailed yesterday do not prevail today, and those which prevail today will not prevail tomorrow. This law seems to have universal application.

In the field of health care, there seems to be a constantly-changing list of "popular" human maladies. It is as though we have a need to suffer. This "need" is opportunistic and will use, to its end, any new maladies which become available. New maladies are discovered by health care professionals and researchers, and popularized by newspapers, television and tabloids sold at supermarket checkout lines. A potentially fruitful area of research, with great implications for the health care industry, is the underlying basis for this "need to suffer."

I entered the general practice of osteopathic medicine and surgery in 1964. It didn't take long to assemble a list of health disorders which fulfilled patients' "need to suffer." Peptic ulcer was for aspiring and successful business executives. Depression and menstrual problems (often treated by a hysterectomy) were for unfulfilled and creatively frustrated housewives. Hemorrhoids were for blue collar workers and "macho" types. Obesity could be used to demonstrate financial success, as a means to obtain amphetamines and other "uppers" for appetite control or as a defense against unwanted sexual approaches. There were various "pain syndromes" which could be used by the guilt-ridden and the martyrs. These pain syndromes did not seem to involve the head as much then as they do now.

The 1980's have brought changes in the popularity list. Twenty years ago a pocketful of antacids (probably Maalox) marked you as a highly intelligent, upwardly mobile American success story. Today, the same personality type will probably have to show a coronary bypass scar in order to prove his success. I say "his" because women have not gotten into the coronary-bypass game nearly as much as men. Women instead display their oral appliances and splints, the badge of the "TMJ syndrome," a most popular female malady.

Probably the second most popular women's condition in this decade (taking over the position previously held by hypoglycemia) is candidiasis. This relates to more generalized debility, depression and pain (as did hypoglycemia). The pain is not usually as focused as it is in the TMJ syndrome.

Personally, I believe that had the TMJ syndrome enjoyed its present level of popularity while Hans Selye was doing his stress research, he might have discussed the "quadrad of stress" rather than the "triad of stress" (peptic ulcer, heart disease and adrenal dysfunction).

I do not want to imply that there is no such thing as valid TMJ syndrome or candidiasis. I do say that these conditions have become "fad" or "waste basket" diagnoses which are grossly overused.

The TMJ syndrome is not new. It was originally called "Costen's syndrome." Costen, an allopathic physician who specialized in otorhinolaryngology, published a description of the syndrome in 1936 (COSTEN). He described the syndrome as consisting of: (1) disturbed temporomandibular joint function involving pain, lack of mobility, noise (clicking and crepitus) and sometimes swelling; (2) secondary neuralgias such as facial pain, pain at the vertex of the skull, pain around the ears and a burning sensation involving the mucosa of the nose, throat and sometimes the tongue; (3) secondary ear symptoms such as tinnitus (ringing), hearing loss and feelings of congestion in the ears, usually due to dysfunction of the auditory tubes; and (4) less frequently, herpetiform lesions of the external ear canal, the mucosa of the mouth and/or the tongue, complaints of dizziness, dry mouth and nystagmus.

Costen estimated that 85% of patients with this syndrome were suffering from dental malocclusion causing temporomandibular joint deterioration and dysfunction. He attributed the other 15% of cases to bruxism and emotional causes.

In my professional life, I have the privilege of discussing health, health problems and disease with many patients, non-patient laypersons, and health care professionals. I would like to share some comments and opinions from health care professionals about the TMJ syndrome.

- A dentist specializing in temporomandibular joint problems stated that the self-help techniques which are described in chapter 12 and appendix G of my first book (UPLEDGER 1983) were more effective than his splints; he now uses the self-help techniques exclusively. These techniques (reviewed in section VII) are also taught in our workshops.
- Another dentist now uses only craniosacral therapy, biofeedback and psychotherapy. He feels that the TMJ syndrome is usually a result of craniosacral system dysfunction and/or tension and emotional stress. He prefers to treat the cause rather than the effect.
- Another dentist feels that the temporomandibular joint problem is primary in less than 10% of the patients referred to him.
- Another dentist now feels that craniosacral decompression therapy, better nutrition for the joint and its adnexa and time would heal over 90% of the problems he sees.
- Another dentist has reduced his splint usage by over 50% in just a few months since he was introduced to craniosacral therapeutic decompression of the joint.
- An osteopathic physician treating temporomandibular joint problems through a combination of craniosacral therapy and self-help techniques reports no failures (as yet).

The list goes on. Many dentists, medical doctors, osteopaths and physiotherapists have reported excellent results with TMJ syndrome using the techniques mentioned above in various combinations.

Our own experience, as we search for underlying causes of temporomandibular joint problems, has been very positive. Our approach includes the mobilization and balancing of the temporal bones, the related membrane system, the mandible and the temporomandibular joints themselves; we combine these techniques with stress management and psychotherapy. We have found that the temporomandibular joint possesses remarkable ability to adapt and reconstruct, given the chance. A minority of cases require occlusal work (involving mandibular splints and focused primarily on the vertical bite dimension); this is done after the craniosacral system is considered sufficiently functional and while stress and emotional problems are being treated. In our opinion, over-correction by splinting which is too directive may interfere with natural adaptive and healing processes. Our goal is to decompress the joints, balance the craniosacral system and let Nature take its course.

The temporomandibular joint is apparently quite resistant to arthritis. In fact, arthritis of various types probably accounts for less than 5% of true temporomandibular joint problems. Post-traumatic calcium deposits, fractures which have healed in abnormal position, disc resorption, atrophy of the mandibular condyle and/or glenoid fossa and malignant changes also account for a small number of temporomandibular joint dysfunctions.

Masseteric hypertrophy syndrome should be mentioned at this time. This syndrome, which may be familial, congenital or acquired, involves a benign hypertrophy of the masseter muscle on one or both sides. This hypertrophy gives the misleading appearance of a parotid tumor which on X-ray may appear to involve the mandible. The mandible, over time, responds to the chronic pull upon it by flaring laterally at its inferior border where the hypertrophic muscle attaches.

II. STRUCTURE OF THE TEMPOROMANDIBULAR JOINT

A. Introduction

The temporomandibular joints are unique in that they are paired joints which connect the same bone (the mandible) to symmetrically paired skull bones (the temporals). Thus, to be functional, the joints must work in reasonable synchrony. If one of the two becomes dysfunctional for any reason, it automatically influences and stresses the other.

The joints are symmetric and generally ellipsoidal in shape. The larger arc is provided by the fossa of the temporal bone. There is a temporal eminence (bony prominence) at the anterior end of each fossa. These eminences (discussed further in section VI) are frequently a source of dysfunction.

Each temporomandibular joint is synovial, containing two cavities which under normal circumstances do *not* communicate. There is a fibroarticular disc separating the two cavities, and functionally dividing each temporomandibular joint into two joints. The upper joint (gliding/arthrodial type) is between the disc and the temporal bone; the lower joint (hinge/ginglymoid type) is between the disc and the mandibular condyle. This subdivision allows for functional versatility, the necessity for which will become evident as our discussion continues (ILLUSTRATION 3-1).

B. Joint classifications

Joints are areas of contact between bones, usually permitting movement. There are many systems for classifying joints; none is totally satisfactory. Perhaps the most widely used is the Nomina Anatomica system, which classifies joints according to the types of tissue which separate the ends of the involved bones, i.e., fibrous, cartilaginous and synovial joints.

1. Fibrous joints are those in which the bone ends nearly contact each other, being separated only by a thin layer of fibrous tissue. These joints allow very little movement. Examples (representing three subtypes) are the sutures between the flat bones of the cranial vault, the joint between a tooth and the maxilla or mandible and the joint between the distal ends of the tibia and fibula (ILLUSTRATION 3-2-A).

INSET

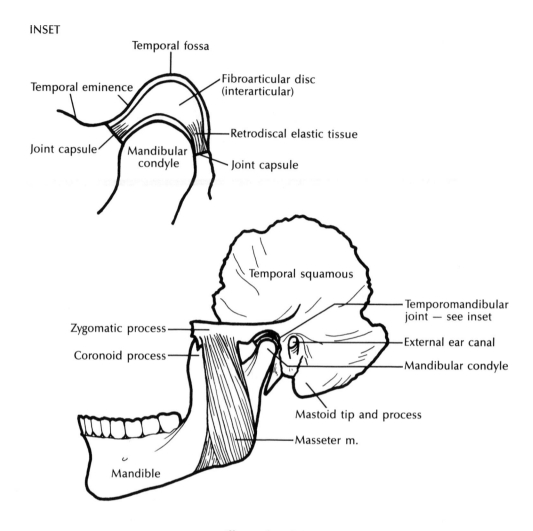

Illustration 3-1
Major Components of the Temporomandibular Joint

2. In cartilaginous joints, the bone ends are joined by hyaline cartilage or a fibrocartilage disc. Examples of the subtype (synchondrosis) involving hyaline cartilage are the spheno-occipital joint (where some movement is possible) and the union of the ilium/ischium/pubis to form the acetabulum. Examples of the subtype (symphysis) involving a fibrocartilage disc are the symphysis pubis and the joints between vertebral bodies. There is usually a thin layer of hyaline cartilage between the disc and bone in this subtype, and limited movement is possible (ILLUSTRATION 3-2-B).

3. Synovial joints are the most complex in design and allow the most freedom of movement. Most of the joints in the arms and legs are of this type. The integrity of synovial joints depends on the connective tissue of the capsule, and on surrounding ligaments and muscles. The contiguous bone surfaces are covered by hyaline

1 — INTERPARIETAL SUTURE
(TOP VIEW)

2 — TIBIOFIBULAR JOINT OF THE ANKLE
(FRONT VIEW)

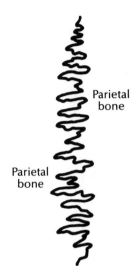

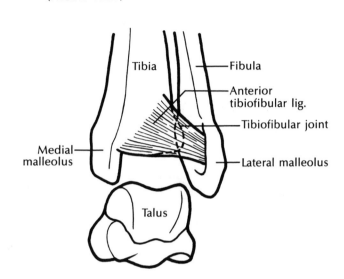

Illustration 3-2-A
Examples of Fibrous Joints

1 — SYMPHYSIS PUBIS
(CORONAL SECTION)

2 — SPHENOBASILAR SYNCHONDROSIS
(SAGGITAL SECTION)

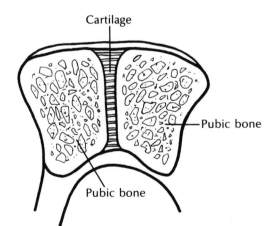

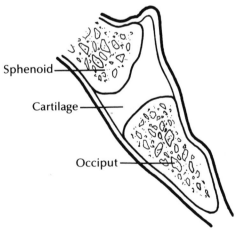

Illustration 3-2-B
Examples of Cartilagenous Joints

cartilage; the joint cavity is lined by a synovial membrane which produces a viscous lubricating fluid (synovial fluid) (ILLUSTRATION 3-2-C).

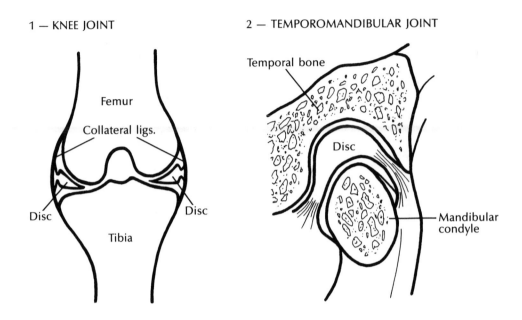

1 — KNEE JOINT   2 — TEMPOROMANDIBULAR JOINT

Illustration 3-2-C
Examples of Synovial Joints

Some synovial joint cavities (e.g., in the temporomandibular joint) are wholly divided by an articular disc. Some (e.g., the knee) are partially divided by a meniscus. These discs and menisci are made of fibrocartilage and are not attached to the bones. The nonarticular surfaces of the discs are covered by synovial membrane; the articular surfaces are not.

Synovial joints are classified into subtypes according to their anatomic design. Several subtypes are briefly described below.

Hinge (uniaxial) joints are designed to permit movement in one plane only. Examples are the elbow and interphalangeal joints of the fingers and toes.

Pivot (trochoid) joints involve bones oriented around a longitudinal axis and allowing rotation. There is typically a ring of ligamentous tissue restricting movement other than rotation. An example is the axis-atlas joint, in which the dens (upward projection of the axis) is surrounded by the anterior arch of the atlas and a transverse ligament (ILLUSTRATION 3-3). The proximal joint between radius and ulna is also classified as a pivot.

Condyloid joints allow motion in more than one plane; some allow a combination of rotation and axial motion. This is a broad classification including most of the synovial joints not mentioned above.

The temporomandibular joint is complex in that it is divided into two synovial cavities by its disc. It allows "hinge" movement, gliding and limited rotation. One temporomandibular joint cannot move without accommodational movement in its

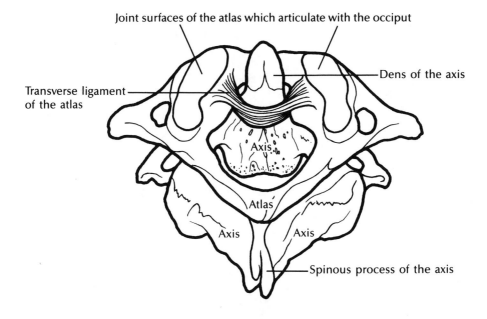

Joint surfaces of the atlas which articulate with the occiput

Dens of the axis

Transverse ligament of the atlas

Axis

Atlas

Axis

Axis

Spinous process of the axis

Illustration 3-3
Superior Posterior View of the Atlanto-Axial Joint

counterpart on the other side because the mandible, the primary bone involved (accommodational movement by the temporals is slight), is a single bone.

C. Components of the temporomandibular joint

1. Temporal joint surface. The temporomandibular joint surface of the temporal bone is usually less than 2.5cm long. It is oriented in an approximately transverse plane. Posteriorly, it has an arc of about 120⁰, located just in front of the external ear canal. The arc is oriented so that if it were to be almost equally bisected by one of its radii, an extension of that radius would bisect the temporal-parietal suture. Anteriorly, the arc ends at the posterior limit of the temporal articular eminence, where the direction of the arc is reversed. The eminence has its apex aimed inferiorly and a posterior slope varying between 30⁰ and 60⁰ from horizontal. The appearance of the eminence plus the arc of the joint fossa can best be described as an "S" lying on its side (ILLUSTRATION 3-4).

This joint surface is not covered by hyaline cartilage, but rather by dense fibrous tissue, which improves the potential for regeneration and remodeling of the joint surface and reduces the risk of degenerative arthritic change. Just beneath the fibrous layer, and protected by it, is a layer of proliferative (growth) cartilage providing for rapid bone growth and remodeling.

2. Mandibular condyle. The condyle may be likened to a transversely oriented cylinder seated atop the posterior part of the ramus. It measures about 2cm from side

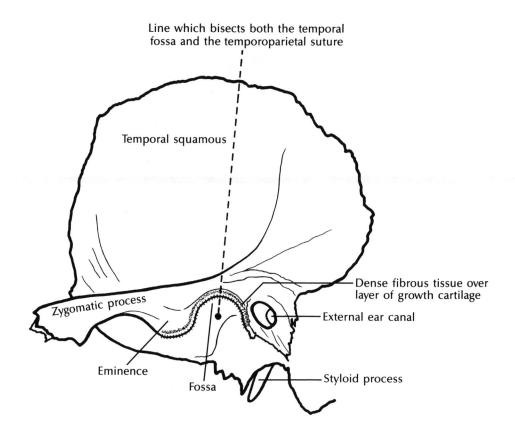

Line which bisects both the temporal fossa and the temporoparietal suture

Temporal squamous

Dense fibrous tissue over layer of growth cartilage

External ear canal

Zygomatic process

Styloid process

Eminence

Fossa

Illustration 3-4
Lateral View of Temporal Bone

to side and 1cm from front to back. The temporomandibular joint surface of the condyle consists of layers of dense fibrous tissue and proliferative cartilage similar to those of the temporal surface. Between the proliferative layer and the deeper bone tissue is a layer of hyaline cartilage also capable of producing bony matrix (an ability not usually seen in hyaline cartilage). This tissue modification makes the condyle more adaptable; most temporomandibular joint remodeling occurs at the condylar surface rather than the temporal surface (ILLUSTRATION 3-5).

3. Interarticular disc. The disc of the temporomandibular joint has been described (often by surgeons) as incapable of remodeling (REES 1954; SICHER 1944). I would hesitate to make such a statement until cases have been observed in which the disc has been given optimal opportunity to reconstruct itself.

The disc is of variable histologic composition; it is mostly fibrous tissue but may contain up to 40% cartilage. It is essentially an oval plate thicker posteriorly than anteriorly. This helps to prevent the disc from moving too far forward and losing its interposition between the condyle and temporal bone; it also helps move the disc

CUT AWAY TOP VIEW OF CONDYLE

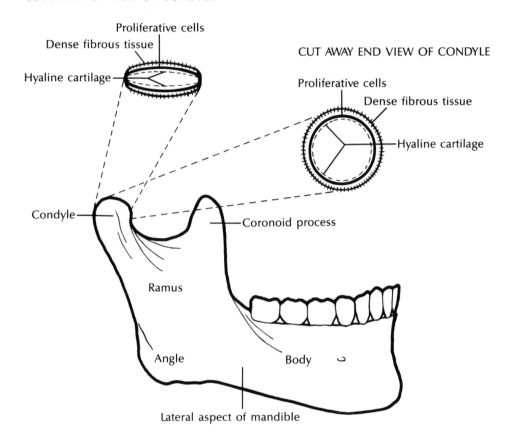

Illustration 3-5
Mandibular Condyle

backward when the joint is compressed by chewing or clenching of the jaws. Its shape is such that it accommodates the articular surfaces of both the temporal and condyle.

The circumference of the disc is attached to the joint capsule either directly or indirectly through connective tissue. Anteriorly, the disc is connected to the tendon of the superior portion of the lateral pterygoid muscle, contraction of which moves the disc forward. Posteriorly, this movement is opposed by the disc's attachment to the retrodiscal tissue (SECTION II.D), which acts reciprocally with the superior lateral pterygoid so that when the muscle relaxes the retrodiscal tissue pulls the disc backward, like a rubber band. As a result, the disc remains in place between the condyle and temporal joint surface. Loss of elasticity in the retrodiscal tissue accounts for many disc problems. Rest, improved nutrition and decompression of this elastic tissue will often result in its revitalization and some return of elastic function. It is apparent that learned relaxation of the lateral pterygoid is essential in order to rest the retrodiscal tissue; biofeedback training can help.

Medially and laterally, the disc is secured to the medial and lateral poles of the condyle by tough fibrous bands called collateral ligaments, which allow the disc to move forward and backward in hinge fashion over the cylindrically shaped and transversely oriented condyle. The disc remains interposed between the condyle and temporal bone as the condyle glides back and forth over the surfaces of the temporal fossa and temporal eminence. For normal temporomandibular joint function, the disc must always be interposed in this way; TMJ syndrome occurs when it moves elsewhere (ILLUSTRATION 3-6).

SAGITTAL SECTION THROUGH DISC

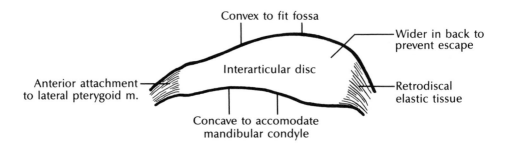

LATERAL VIEW   TOP VIEW

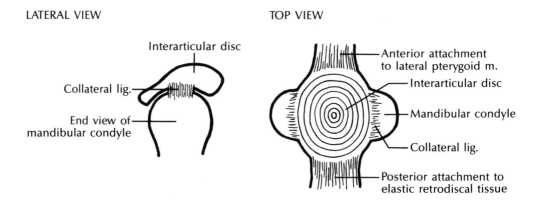

Illustration 3-6
Interarticular Disc

The disc is composed of concentrically arranged fibers and is thicker peripherally than at the center. It may even perforate at the center, in which case communication is established between the two fluid-filled synovial cavities, which are normally separated. I do not know the functional significance of the separation, nor the clinical implications (if any) of its loss.

The disc is moderately flexible but not normally compressible. It is vascular, contains sensory receptors and innervation and sends signals to the brain when it is suffering unusual stress or compression. It also sends proprioceptive information which is integrated into the trigeminal system, facilitating decisions on how hard to bite down.

The disc moves on the condyle around a transverse axis passing through the two poles of the condyle. This axis is located near the anterior margin of the foramen magnum. We may think of the disc-condyle complex as a functional unit articulating with the temporal fossa and eminence, and gliding over the articular surface of the temporal bone (the condyle moving from front to back) as we open and close the jaw. This gliding is necessary because the actual axis of rotation of the mandible is 3-5cm below the condyle (ILLUSTRATION 3-7).

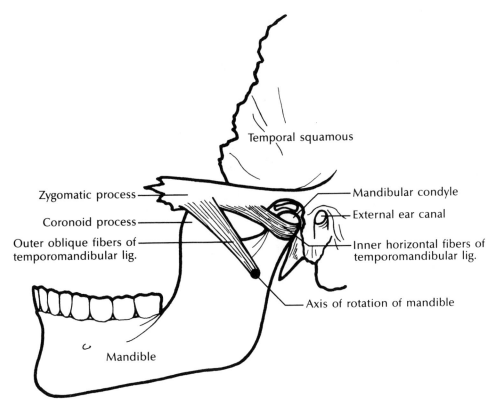

Illustration 3-7
Temporomandibular Ligament

Several factors are mandatory for normal disc function: (1) normal and relatively undamaged and symmetrical bony surfaces on both sides of the head; (2) good synovial fluid lubrication; (3) good proprioceptive information to prevent unusual compression of the disc as a result of inadequate or unintentionally hard clenching of the teeth; and (4) occlusion should be such that maximal intercuspation does not produce a sliding at the end point of each power closure of the jaw. Malocclusion may cause movement in the temporomandibular joint when maximum compression of the joint occurs, resulting in friction wear and tear on the joint.

D. Temporomandibular joint capsule and soft tissue contents

The temporomandibular joint capsule is a thin, fibrous envelope which attaches above to the circumference of the articulating surface of the temporal, below to the neck of the condyle and in between to the circumference of the interarticular disc. It is well vascularized and pain-sensitive; its connection to the nervous system is via the trigeminal system, specifically the auriculotemporal, masseteric and posterior deep temporal branches.

The portion of the capsule above the disc has a loose, bellowy structure which allows the gliding movement of the disc-condyle complex forward and backward over the temporal joint surface. Below the disc, the capsule is rather taut since the disc moves closely with the mandible. Synovial fluid secreted inside the compartments lubricates the joint, supplies some nutrition, carries waste metabolites away, acts as a medium for phagocyte movement and keeps the capsule inflated to its proper shape.

The retrodiscal tissue (SECTION II.C.3) completes the separation of the intracapsular space into two separate cavities. This structure is composed of loose connective tissue attached to the posterior aspect of the disc and the inner surface of the posterior capsule. It is well-vascularized and innervated, and is covered by a fluid-secreting synovial membrane. When the disc is in its forward-most position, the retrodiscal tissue is stretched to its extreme and acts to stabilize the disc.

The retrodiscal tissue is divided into upper and lower laminae. The upper lamina possesses the elastic quality which opposes the pull of the lateral pterygoid. The lower lamina is mainly non-elastic and serves to limit the extreme forward movement of the disc; it attaches to the posterior disc surface and to the posterior condyle of the mandible just below the margin of the articular surface, and thus limits the anterior hinge movement of the disc on the condyle.

E. Other ligaments

You can easily locate the axis of rotation of your own mandible by gently palpating the angle and ramus of the mandible as you slowly open and close your jaw. With a little exploration, the transverse axial pivot point is easily found. Locating this axis of rotation will help you understand the functions of the following ligaments and of the temporomandibular joint system.

1. The **temporomandibular ligament** strengthens the antero-lateral part of the temporomandibular joint capsule; it is actually a localized thickening of the capsule. Above, it is firmly attached to the zygomatic process of the temporal. From this attachment, it divides into inner horizontal and outer oblique portions. The inner horizontal fibers run from the zygomatic process to the lateral pole of the condyle and act to prevent posterior dislocation (the condyle moving too far backward when the mouth is closed). The outer oblique fibers run from the zygomatic process diagonally downward and posteriorly to attach to the neck of the ramus. These fibers cause the condyle to move forward when the mouth is opened. It is largely because of this ligament that the transverse axis of rotation of the mandible (when opening or closing the mouth) is located in the ramus or even lower in the angle of that bone (ILLUSTRATION 3-7). This protects the tissues just posterior to the ramus from compression injury when the mouth is opened widely. The ligament also protects against posterior and inferior dislocation of the jaw.

Each temporomandibular ligament is about 3cm long and 1-2cm wide, broadening posteriorly. It is covered by tissue of the parotid gland, and the horizontal part attaches to the poles of the condyle together with the lateral collateral ligaments of the interarticular disc.

2. The **sphenomandibular ligament** is a (bilateral) thin, flat, fibrous band, about 2-3cm long and 0.5cm wide, oriented vertically and connecting the spines of the sphenoid with the internal aspect of the lower ramus of the mandible. It attaches on the ramus somewhat anteriorly to the temporomandibular joint capsule, and acts to vertically suspend the mandible from the sphenoid. It widens somewhat as it descends (ILLUSTRATION 3-8).

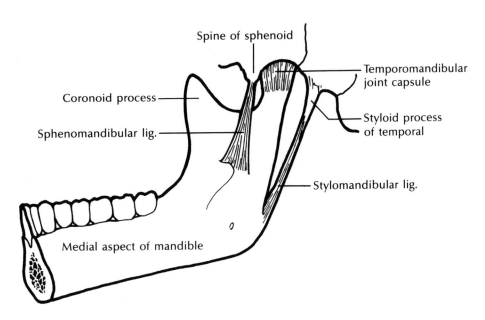

Illustration 3-8
Suspensory Ligaments of the Mandible

Several important structures pass between this ligament and the mandible. From above, we encounter the lateral pterygoid muscle, the auriculo-temporal nerve, the maxillary artery and vein, the inferior alveolar artery, vein, nerve and some lobules of the parotid gland. The ligament runs between the lateral and medial pterygoid muscles. It is therefore related to the medial pterygoid medially, as well as the levator veli palatini muscle and the pharyngeal wall.

The sphenomandibular ligament develops embryologically from Meckel's cartilage, which is part of the mandibular arch. It is common to find some fibers from the ligament penetrating the petrotympanic fissure, entering the middle ear and attaching to the malleus (one of the tiny bones attached to the eardrum). Problems with the ligament can therefore result in hearing impairment or tinnitus.

3. The **stylomandibular ligament** is actually a specialized band of cervical fascia. It connects the styloid process of the temporal with the posterior aspect of the mandibular angle, and helps separate the submaxillary and parotid glands. It also provides partial origin for some of the fibers of the styloglossus muscle which extends upward into the tongue. The styloid process parallels the posterior belly of the digastric muscle (SECTION III.E.5.a) (ILLUSTRATION 3-8).

Obviously, disruption of the interconnections of the mandible, sphenoid and temporal bones via these ligaments can compromise craniosacral system function.

F. Developmental considerations

The structure of the temporomandibular joint is unique to mammals and arose during the evolutionary transition between reptiles and mammals. In reptiles, the jaw joint is between bones which are analogous to the middle ear bones in humans. During human fetal development, the jaw joint moves from the ear to its position in front of the ear (ontogeny recapitulating phylogeny). Frequently, the lateral pterygoid muscle sends fibers through the interarticular disc and into the ear, attaching to the malleus. This attachment persists throughout adult life, another example of the association between jaw function and hearing.

After we are born, the temporomandibular joint moves upward in relation to the "biteline" between the teeth, until at maturity the joint is usually more than an inch higher than the biteline. Before we begin to chew, the temporomandibular joint surfaces are heavily innervated and vascularized; they become less so as time goes by. Perhaps feedback from the joint surfaces early in life teaches us to chew safely, and the habit persists throughout life.

As the teeth appear and the level of the temporomandibular joint rises in relation to the biteline, the structure and function of the masticatory system are modified. If this system appears dysfunctional in some cases, perhaps it is attempting to adapt to an external force or problem. If this is the case, dental occlusal work may be counterproductive. It seems better to me to consider all external factors before performing occlusal or other invasive work. I have one patient whose bite improved in response to Alexander work, which corrected the posture. Another patient's temporomandibular joint and occlusal problems were "spontaneously healed" when we released the abnormal contracture of the right piriformis muscle.

III. MUSCLES

A. Temporalis muscle

1. Introduction. During my tenure at the Michigan State University College of Osteopathic Medicine, most of my time was spent as a clinical researcher in the Department of Biomechanics. I had frequent opportunity to dissect heads of non-human primate species, and was continually amazed at the thickness and bulk of the temporalis muscle in baboons. Clearly, these animals can bite with much greater force than we can, as one would expect based on their environment and dietary habits. In humans, increased tonus of the temporalis is often correlated with high levels of emotional stress. Hypertrophy of this muscle or the masseter is more likely to be related to temporomandibular joint problems than with enhanced chewing force.

2. Anatomy. The temporalis has an extensive origin, arising from the external surfaces of all the bones making up the temporal fossa on the side of the skull. It also has some origin from the superficial fasciae which cover its lateral aspects.

The temporal fossa is oval in shape, measuring approximately 10cm from front to back, and 7cm from top to bottom. It is bounded anteriorly by the processes which unite the zygomatic and frontal bones; its oval boundary from the root of the frontal's zygomatic process is marked by a ridge of bone called the superior temporal line. This line, in lateral view, closely parallels the silhouette of the head (ILLUSTRATION 3-9).

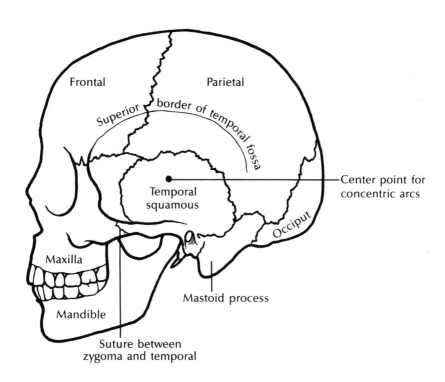

Illustration 3-9
Boundaries of the Temporal Fossa

This boundary line defines the periphery of the origin of the temporalis muscle, which occupies about one third of the lateral skull. From its anterior origin, the superior temporal line travels in a posterior and slightly superior direction across the lateral part of the coronal suture to the parietal bone, then levels off to a horizontal direction and begins curving downward about 4-5cm past its coronal suture crossing. Thus, it describes a half circle whose centerpoint would be on the temporal-parietal suture above the external ear canal opening. It then travels downward and anteriorly, achieving an almost horizontal orientation when it finally blends into the root of the zygomatic process of the temporal bone.

The lateral wall of the temporal fossa is composed of the zygomatic arch of the temporal bone and the superficial fasciae which overlie the fossa. The deep wall is formed by the external surface of the great wing of the sphenoid, the lateral surfaces of the frontal bone and parietal bones below the superior temporal line and the squamous surface of the temporal bone.

The fibers of the temporalis are arranged as though they are radii diverging from the coronoid process of the mandible toward the periphery of the temporal fossa. Fibers from the anterior parts of the fossa generally connect the frontal and sphenoid bones to their insertions on the coronoid process.

Fibers arising from the part of the temporal fossa posterior to the coronal suture converge onto a tendon which passes beneath the zygomatic arch and attaches (mostly medially) to the coronoid process and ramus of the mandible as far down as the root of the third molar (ILLUSTRATION 3-10).

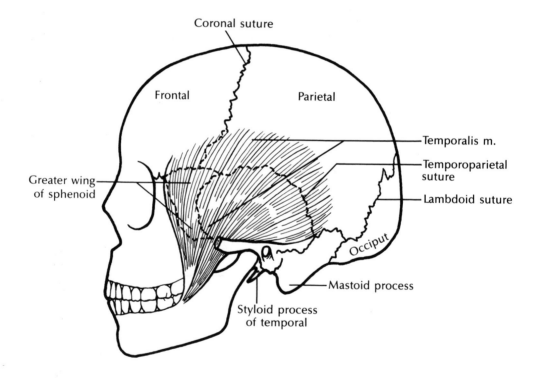

Illustration 3-10
Temporalis Muscle (Note Divergence of Fibers)

The temporal fascia is a very strong sheet of fibrous connective tissue (actually an extension of the deep cervical fascia) covering the temporalis and providing attachment for some of the muscle fibers. Above, it attaches to the superior temporal line to form a superior closure for the temporal fossa, and is continuous with the pericranium which covers the external surface of the bones of the cranial vault above the line.

Below, it attaches to the internal and external surfaces of the zygomatic arch, where it is continuous with the masseter fascia.

3. Action. There are several important principles of action of the temporalis which must be considered in relation to the temporomandibular joint. First, it is probable that the temporalis has the ability to contract only a specific subset of its fibers at a given time. That is, the anterior, middle or posterior parts of the muscle might contract independently of each other in order to create force in different directions. Second, the axis of rotation of the mandible is down on the ramus or even the angle. Thus, the condyle-disc complex is forced to glide forward and backward on the temporal surface of the joint to accommodate the opening and closing of the jaw. This axis location results in leverage between the temporalis and the coronoid process which gives the temporalis a significant mechanical advantage during chewing and biting (ILLUSTRATION 3-11).

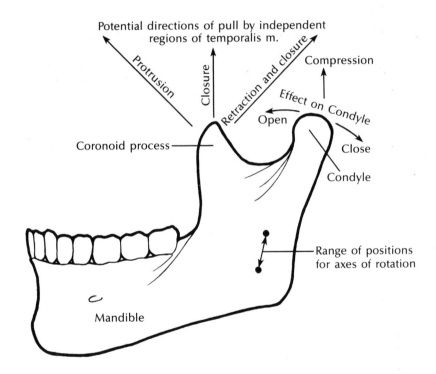

Illustration 3-11
Effects of Temporalis Muscle on Mandible

Because of its broad origin, the temporalis can do several things. Contraction of its anterior fibers moves the coronoid process superiorly. Because of the location of the axis of rotation of the mandible, this causes the condyle to move posteriorly on the temporal surface of the joint. Contraction of its middle fibers closes the mandible and simultaneously elevates the condyle and ramus. This compresses the temporomandibular joint in a more superior and posterior direction. Contraction of its posterior fibers (which insert via tendon principally on the medial ramus and angle) raises the mandible into the temporomandibular joint fossa on the temporal bone with a more posteriorly-directed force, which can result in joint impaction or compression. As the anterior fibers contract, they tend to immobilize the sphenoid and frontal bones. As the middle fibers contract, they tend to shear the temporoparietal suture and force the parietal bones to favor a position of medial compression or internal rotation. This tension on the parietals favors an extension habitus of the cranial vault which is transmitted to the cranial base. Selective contraction of the posterior fibers pulls the posterolateral aspects of the parietal and temporal forward and down, which favors cranial vault flexion and forcibly retracts the mandible.

The temporalis muscle also has the ability to cause a shearing dysfunction of the temporoparietal suture (UPLEDGER 1983, CHAPTER 12) because the suture is beveled sharply in relation to the surface of the skull. The bevel direction, in coronal section, is from superior-lateral to inferior-medial. Since the temporalis muscle attaches to the parietal bone above the suture and to the coronoid process of the mandible below, contraction of the middle part of the muscle first clenches the teeth. When the mandible is completely closed, further contraction of the muscle compresses the temporomandibular joint. This compression fixes the temporal bone to the mandible so that further contraction of the muscle causes a downward pull on the parietal against the temporal bone, and a resultant shearing force across the temporoparietal suture (ILLUSTRATION 3-12). When this condition is chronic, sutural dysfunction results. The condition can be produced by ongoing emotional stress and/or loss of vertical dimension of the bite. In the latter case, when the temporalis contracts, the molars do not meet soon enough and the shearing force is created by the sequence of events described above (UPLEDGER 1983, APPENDIX G).

4. Clinical. One can easily see the relationships among the craniosacral system, temporalis muscle and temporomandibular joint.

Suppose that the temporalis on one side is hypertonic (or hypotonic) and the other is not. This can occur for many reasons: neurogenic origin; less vertical dimension of the teeth on one side; habitual chewing on one side; previous trauma to the mandible or side of the head; or a cranial base side-bending problem (which may arise from as far away as the sacrum).

Treatment of the temporomandibular joint as an isolated entity addresses only the surface of the problem. In my experience, TMJ syndrome is more often a symptom than a cause. True, the symptom may require specific treatment, but to treat only the temporomandibular joint dysfunction is to invite eventual failure of treatment. The joint is part of a whole person. Its dysfunction usually signifies that something else is wrong.

5. Innervation to the temporalis comes from the trigeminal system via temporal branches from the anterior trunk of its mandibular division. These nerves usually pass between the upper origin of the lateral pterygoid muscle and the sphenoid and temporal bones which form the margin of the infratemporal fossa, located below and medial to the zygomatic arch. The foramen ovale and foramen spinosum open into this fossa, as do the inferior orbital fissure and pterygomaxillary fissure. Structures passing through this fossa include the mandibular and maxillary nerves, maxillary blood vessels,

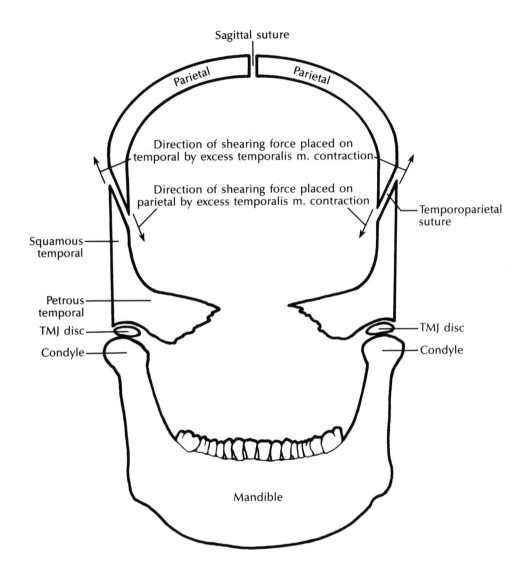

Illustration 3-12
Mechanics of Sutural Strain from Excess
Temporalis Muscle Contraction

pterygoid venous plexus and parts of the temporalis and medial/lateral pterygoid muscles. The temporal nerves may also pass between the two heads of the lateral pterygoid.

The nerves are usually accompanied by the deep temporal arteries which branch from the internal maxillary artery. Before entering the temporal bone, the nerves and arteries travel upward between the muscle and the bone for an inch or more, then unite on the outer surface of the lateral pterygoid.

Considering the fact that the trigeminal nerve is related to the reticular alarm system (RAS) in the central nervous system, and that the RAS is activated by danger, anger, etc., it seems reasonable that activation of this alarm system is often expressed via the trigeminal system in the muscles of mastication, the largest of which is the temporalis.

B. Masseter muscle

1. Mandibular sling. The masseter and medial pterygoid muscles are spoken of collectively as the mandibular sling because they suspend the angle of the mandible in a "sling" of muscle and fascia. This sling actually forms a maxillary-mandibular joint in the functional sense, with the temporomandibular joint acting as a guide. The axis of rotation of the joint is determined by this muscular sling, in conjunction with the sphenomandibular and temporomandibular ligaments. The muscles making up the mandibular sling work together to close the jaw and prevent inferior dislocation of the temporomandibular joint.

2. Structure and function. The masseter muscle (which forms the external component of the sling) is divided into three parts: superficial, intermediate and deep. The superficial part originates from the anterior two-thirds of the lower border of the zygomatic arch, the intermediate part from the anterior two-thirds of the inner surface of the arch and the deep part from the posterior one-third of the inner surface of the arch. Some fibers of the deep part may arise from the temporalis fascia or from the temporalis itself. The origins of the intermediate and deep parts on the zygomatic arch are continuous with each other. The superficial part of the muscle overlies the intermediate part, then runs downward and posteriorly so that it covers the deep part by the time it is halfway between the zygomatic arch and the inferior mandibular border. Blending of the three parts begins as they extend inferiorly, and is complete by the time they are within 2.5cm of their common insertion. This insertion almost completely covers the lateral surface of the mandibular ramus from 2.5cm below the condylar and coronoid processes down to the inferior margin of the angle (ILLUSTRATION 3-13).

The masseteric nerve enters the deep surface of the muscle, with the associated artery and vein, by passing through the mandibular notch. The nerve is a branch of the mandibular division of the trigeminal system. The artery is a branch of the maxillary artery after it passes between the lateral pterygoid and temporalis muscles. The masseter muscle is crossed by the parotid duct and by branches of the facial nerve; problems with the muscle may affect either of these structures. "Masseteric hypertrophy syndrome," in which the muscle is greatly enlarged and may be mistaken for a tumor, was mentioned in section I.

3. The **parotid-masseteric fascia** covers the external surface of the masseter. It divides into lamina in order to envelop the parotid gland, which lies partially external to the masseter. The upper end of this fascia is attached to the zygomatic arch. Posteriorly, it is continuous with the investing fascia of the sternocleidomastoid muscle and attaches to the ramus, such that sternocleidomastoid action influences the mobility of the mandible directly through the fascia. Inferiorly and anteriorly, the fascia attaches to the mandible so that it forms an envelope for the masseter. This envelope is not "sealed," i.e., it is open superiorly where it communicates with the space inside the enclosure of the temporalis fascia. Where the fascia forms the three closed sides of

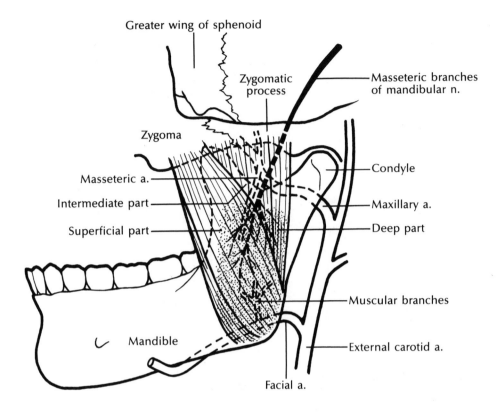

Illustration 3-13
Masseter Muscle

the envelope at its mandibular attachments, it is continuous with the fascia of the medial pterygoid muscle, which is deep to the ramus. Laterally, the masseteric fascia fuses with the superficial fascia by numerous septa which pass through the parotid gland and the envelope formed by the two fasciae. Because of these septa, the parotid gland is not easily dislodged from its compartment as is the submaxillary gland. On the deep side and over the posterior aspect of the ramus, the masseteric fascia is also continuous with the fascia of the posterior digastric muscle. Here it thickens and gets very tough along a line which becomes the stylomandibular ligament (SECTION II.E.3).

An interesting clinical observation regarding the masseter is that on its anterior border, on a level with the corner of the mouth, is an acupuncture point. This was brought to my attention by Louis Moss, M.D., who was then practicing on Harley Street in London. He very modestly named these bilaterally placed points (which are just anterior to the classical Chinese acupuncture points S-6 [Jiache]) the "Moss miracle points." The insertion of needles here will relax lumbar muscle contracture and usually neutralize "long leg syndrome," also known as "short leg syndrome." The needle should penetrate only the fascia at the anterior edge of the muscle, not the buccal mucosa or the masseter itself. I have used this technique many times to relax lumbar muscle spasm and to quickly differentiate functional from anatomic leg length discrepancy.

C. Medial pterygoid muscle

1. Anatomy. The bilateral medial pterygoid muscle, the other component of the mandibular sling, is located opposite the masseter on the inside of the mandible. Its origin is by two slips: the larger from the lateral pterygoid plate of the sphenoid, the smaller from the pyramidal process of the palatine bone and the tuberosity of the maxilla. The lateral pterygoid muscle passes between these two slips (lateral to the large slip and superior to the small slip) (ILLUSTRATION 3-14).

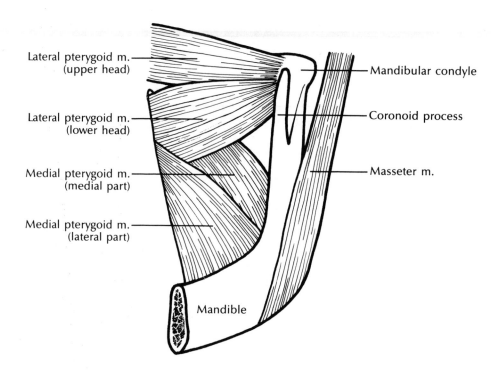

Illustration 3-14
Relationships of Medial and Lateral
Pterygoid Muscles

The insertion of the medial pterygoid muscle is on the inner side of the mandibular angle and ramus as far up as the mandibular foramen, which is located about midway between the mandibular notch and the inferior boundary of the angle. The inferior alveolar nerve and associated vessels pass through this foramen and into the canal which runs within the mandible and communicates with all of the alveolar sockets of the teeth.

Several important structures are located between the upper part of the medial pterygoid and the mandible, including the maxillary blood vessels, inferior alveolar blood vessels, inferior alveolar and lingual nerves and sphenomandibular ligament. At the upper border of the muscle, the chorda tympani nerve joins the lingual nerve. The lingual and inferior alveolar nerves descend across the muscle almost parallel to each other; the lingual is the more anterior of the two. The sphenomandibular ligament

(SECTION II.E.2) attaches to the mandibular lingula, a sharp spiny projection of the mandible anterior to and sometimes circumferentially around the mandibular foramen; this ligament is medial to the vessels and nerves mentioned above.

The medial surface of the medial pterygoid is related to the tensor veli palatini and superior pharyngeal constrictor muscles. The fascia of the medial surface forms one wall of the lateral pharyngeal space (CHAPTER 2, SECTION VI.B.3.c) which surgeons use as an access to the deeper structures of the neck. The lateral surface of the muscle forms the medial boundary of the mandibular space (CHAPTER 2, SECTION VI.B.2.d).

The nerve supply to the medial pterygoid is from a short branch of the mandibular nerve which runs deep to the inferior alveolar and lingual nerves in the mandibular space, and frequently passes (without synapse) through the otic ganglion (CHAPTER 1, SECTION V.H).

2. Pterygoid fascia. This fascia invests both the medial and lateral pterygoid muscles. At its lower borders, along the angle, it is continuous with the masseteric fascia (SECTION III.B.3). It is also continuous with the investing fasciae of the neck below the mandible (CHAPTER 2, SECTION II). All of these fascial systems attach to the mandible, which is therefore subject to forces from several directions. From its mooring on the inferior angle, the pterygoid fascia extends upward and forward to cover the deep surface of the medial pterygoid muscle up to the muscle's origins.

Where the pterygoid fascia attaches to the mandible, it forms an envelope similar to that formed by the masseteric fascia on the outside of the mandible. The medial pterygoid angles away (medially) from the mandible as it ascends; the fascia goes with it and wraps around the muscle to form an investing sheath. In this way, it covers the muscle surface as an envelope after the muscle is no longer attached to the mandible.

On the lateral side of the muscle, the fascia splits to form an envelope which contains the lateral pterygoid muscle. This investing fascia attaches to the infratemporal crest, the inferior part of the lateral sphenoid wing and the lateral surface of the lateral pterygoid plate of the sphenoid (areas of origin for the medial pterygoid). The pterygoid venous plexuses can be seen on the superficial side of the fascia. On the deep side, the pterygoid and temporal fasciae are separated from the buccopharyngeal fascia by a fat pad, an extension of the buccal fat pad.

Between the medial and lateral pterygoids, the fascial sheets attach to the skull. The attachment is on a line between the lateral pterygoid plate and the spine of the sphenoid. Part of this attachment to the spine is where the fascia thickens and forms the sphenomandibular ligament (SECTION II.E.2), which connects the spine to the lingula of the mandible (ILLUSTRATION 3-15).

Another part of the fascia between the two pterygoid muscles forms the pterygospinous ligament, which connects the sphenoid spine to the posterior margin of the lateral pterygoid plate. Sometimes this ligament calcifies, in which case the space between the calcified ligament and the sphenoid body is called the pterygospinous foramen. Whether the ligament is calcified or not, the space formed affords passage to the branches of the mandibular nerve which supply the muscles of mastication (the blood vessels pass between the ramus and the ligament); this nerve emerges from the foramen ovale, located above and slightly posterior to the ligament.

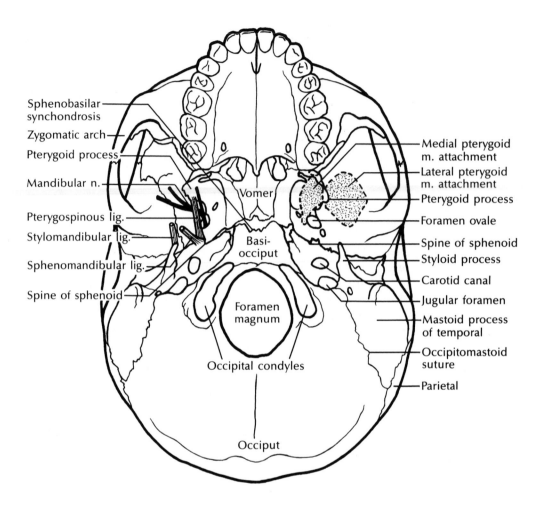

Illustration 3-15
Inferior View of Skull
Showing Connective Tissue Attachments

D. Lateral pterygoid muscle

This muscle runs on an almost horizontal plane, whereas the temporalis, masseter and medial pterygoid muscles are, for the most part, vertically oriented. As the posterior temporalis fibers become more horizontally oriented, they pull backward on the coronoid process; in so doing they act antagonistically to the lateral pterygoid muscle, which pulls the mandibular condyle and its disc forward. The lateral pterygoid muscle seldom acts alone. In conjunction with the medial pterygoid and masseter, it acts to protrude the mandible and lower incisors for biting (e.g., an apple). When these muscles are contracted unilaterally, the mandible is rotated and molar grinding occurs.

The general shape of the lateral pterygoid muscle is conical; the vertical height is greater anteriorly. The muscle originates by two heads. The superior head arises from the infratemporal surface of the great wing of the sphenoid (the roof of the infratemporal fossa) and from the infratemporal crest. The inferior head arises from the lateral surface of the lateral pterygoid plate of the sphenoid.

The muscle is covered on much of its external surface by the pterygoid venous plexus, which passes between the two heads and around the lower border of the muscle such that it extends deep to and between the two pterygoid muscles. The direction of the muscle fibers is generally posterior and lateral; the bones of origin are anterior and medial to the condyles and disc of the temporomandibular joint, where the muscle inserts (ILLUSTRATION 3-16).

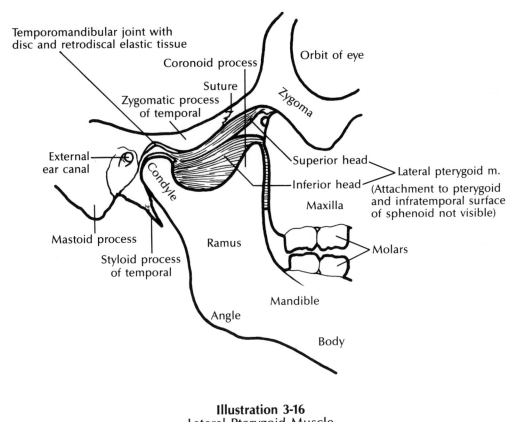

Illustration 3-16
Lateral Pterygoid Muscle

The fibers of the two heads unite as they approach their insertion on the anterior margin of the disc, the capsule and the depression in the anterior neck of the mandible just below the condylar head. The fibers of the superior head remain superior and move the disc and capsule anteriorly when muscular contraction occurs; the retrodiscal tissue (SECTION II.D) returns the disc posteriorly when the superior head of the lateral pterygoid is relaxed. The inferior fibers remain inferior, and insert on the neck of the mandibular condyle. The connection of the lateral pterygoid to the malleus of the middle ear was mentioned in section II.F. During embryological development, the tendon differentiates to form the interarticular disc of the temporomandibular joint.

This connection between the lateral pterygoid, the disc and the middle ear probably helps explain the hearing problems that often accompany TMJ syndrome.

The anatomical relationships of this muscle are numerous, and its dysfunction can produce a variety of symptoms. The mandibular nerve (CHAPTER 1, SECTION IV.D), which supplies all the muscles of mastication, leaves the skull vault through the foramen ovale, which is just deep to the lateral pterygoid muscle. Branches of this nerve include: (1) the masseteric and deep temporalis nerves, which usually pass over the superior head of the lateral pterygoid; (2) the auriculo-temporal nerve, which runs along the deep surface of the superior head; (3) the buccal nerve, which passes between the two heads and then over the surface of the inferior head; (4) the lingual and inferior alveolar nerves, which pass along the deep surface of the two heads, emerge just inferior to the lower border of the muscle, and then travel along the outer surface of the medial pterygoid muscle.

The maxillary artery comes into contact with the lateral pterygoid muscle, sometimes emerging between the two heads to get to the pterygopalatine fossa. The venous plexus which covers the muscle is mentioned above.

The craniosacral balance and release approach to normalization of lateral pterygoid muscle function is essential to the achievement of optimal clinical results in the treatment of TMJ syndrome. Biofeedback and other muscle relaxation techniques are also useful.

E. Accessory muscles of mastication

The muscles to be discussed in this section have no direct relevance to TMJ syndrome or to craniosacral therapy, but I would like to mention them briefly since all are involved in the actions of eating and swallowing (ILLUSTRATION 3-17).

1. Minor lip muscles. The eight muscles listed under a-h below are involved in retracting the lips to get them out of the way during biting movements of the incisors. Muscles a-d are innervated by branches of the facial nerve system, e-h by the facial system and/or the mandibular division of the trigeminal system.

a. The **levator labii superior** raises and protrudes the upper lip. Its origin is from the inferior margin of the orbit of the eye; it inserts into the upper lip bilaterally.

b. The **levator labii superior alaeque nasi** flares the nostrils (to facilitate smelling the food one is about to eat) and assists the levator labii superior in raising the upper lip. It originates from the frontal process of the maxilla and has two insertions: one in the alar cartilage and skin of the nose, the other blending medially with the insertion of the levator labii superior.

c. The **levator anguli oris** raises the corners of the mouth as in smiling, and assists in raising the upper lip. It originates from the canine fossa (just below the infraorbital foramen) and inserts into the corner of the mouth.

d. The **zygomaticus major and minor** raise the upper lip and are involved in smiling and other facial expressions. The zygomaticus major originates anteriorly to

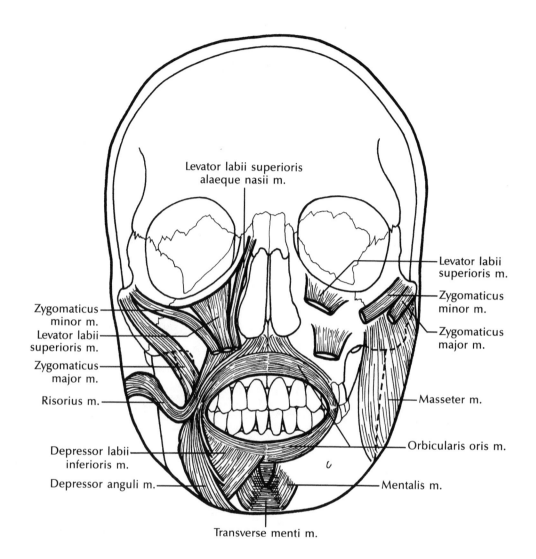

Levator labii superioris
alaeque nasii m.

Levator labii
superioris m.

Zygomaticus
minor m.

Zygomaticus
major m.

Zygomaticus
minor m.

Levator labii
superioris m.

Zygomaticus
major m.

Risorius m.

Masseter m.

Depressor labii
inferioris m.

Orbicularis oris m.

Depressor anguli m.

Mentalis m.

Transverse menti m.

Illustration 3-17
Muscles Which Move the Mouth

the temporozygomatic suture of the zygomatic bone and inserts near the corner of the mouth. The zygomaticus minor originates posteriorly to the zygomatico-maxillary suture and inserts medially to the zygomaticus major.

e. The **risorius** retracts the corners of the mouth in preparation for taking a big bite. It comes from the parotid fascia and inserts into the skin over the corner of the mouth.

f. The **depressor labii inferioris** depresses and protrudes the lower lip. It arises from the anterior mandible between the symphysis menti and mental foramen, and inserts into the skin of the lower lip.

g. The **depressor anguli oris** acts in conjunction (and shares some fibers) with the levator anguli oris to raise or lower the corners of the mouth. It arises from the mandible lateral to the depressor labii inferioris and inserts into the tissue of the angle of the mouth.

h. The **mentalis** is a small conical muscle arising from the mandible anteriorly just below the lower incisors and inserting into the chin tissue. It raises the skin of the chin and thereby helps protrude the lower lip.

2. The **orbicularis oris** brings the lips together after biting and applies them to the lips and gums to assist in control of food position and prevent food from leaving the mouth during chewing. This is a complex muscle with a variety of possible actions, not a simple sphincter around the mouth. It is also involved in speech, whistling, kissing, etc. There are several strata of fibers with different origins (e.g., other facial muscles, bones, other parts of the same muscle) and orientations. Innervation is by the facial system (ILLUSTRATION 3-18).

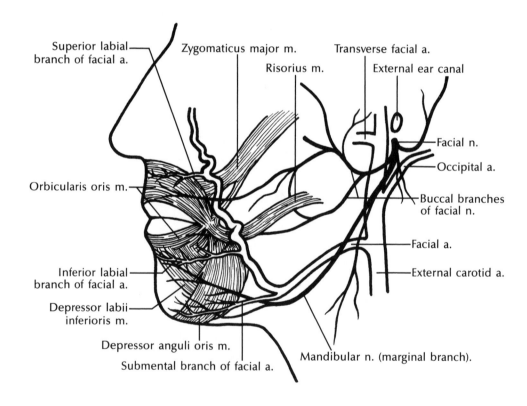

Illustration 3-18
Orbicularis Oris Muscle and Related Structures

3. The **buccinator** (a bilateral muscle) controls the size of the cheek pouches during chewing and is involved in actions such as blowing a trumpet and sucking through a straw. It is quadrilateral in shape and makes up most of the lateral oral cavity. It originates from the alveolar processes of the maxilla and mandible, and posteriorly from the pterygomandibular raphe. This raphe is a band of tough connective tissue extending from the hamulus of the sphenoid's medial pterygoid plate to the posterior external aspect of the mandible at the posterior end of the mylohyoid line. The buccinator inserts, in conjunction with other facial muscles, into the connective tissue and skin around the mouth. Innervation is by the facial system (ILLUSTRATION 3-19).

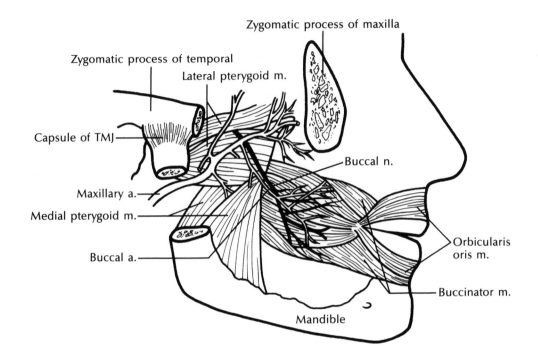

Illustration 3-19
Buccinator Muscle

4. Muscles of the tongue

a. Introduction. The tongue is a complex muscular organ integral to the actions of tasting, chewing, swallowing and speech. It is bisected by a midsagittal septum, i.e., the tongue muscles described below are all paired. The septum extends from the tongue down the anterior wall of the throat and is anchored inferiorly to the hyoid bone.

The muscles of the tongue are classified as extrinsic (having one attachment outside the tongue) (ILLUSTRATIONS 3-20 and 3-21) or intrinsic (attaching at both ends within the tongue itself) (ILLUSTRATION 3-21). The extrinsic muscles act to move the tongue about in the mouth and to protrude it; the intrinsic muscles act primarily to change its shape.

b. The **genioglossus muscle** (extrinsic) originates from a short tendon attached to the superior mental spine of the symphysis menti. This muscle can be compared to a fan, with the tendon as fan handle and the fibers as diverging fan blades. The lower fibers extend down to a connective tissue sheet (aponeurosis) connecting to the hyoid

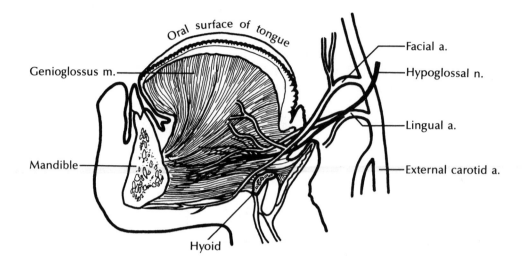

Illustration 3-20
Genioglossus Muscle

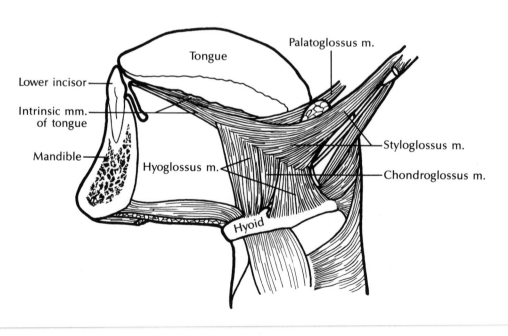

Illustration 3-21
Extrinsic Muscles of the Tongue

bone. The middle and upper fibers fan out to enter the entire undersurface of the tongue (ILLUSTRATION 3-20). A few fibers of the posterior/inferior part may extend into and blend with the middle constrictor muscle of the pharynx. Contraction of the posterior fibers protrudes the tip of the tongue; contraction of the anterior fibers retracts the tongue. Simultaneous bilateral contraction of both sets of fibers shapes the tongue into a channel, allowing one to swallow fluids along the concavity (this is the tongue shape used by infants in suckling).

c. The **hyoglossus muscle** (extrinsic) takes its origin from the length of the greater cornua of the hyoid bone. It passes upward and laterally to enter the tongue. Contraction of this muscle draws the sides of the tongue downward and lowers the tongue in the mouth.

d. The **chondroglossus muscle** (extrinsic) is 2.5cm or less in length. The origin is from the body of the hyoid bone; the insertion is actually a blending with the intrinsic tongue muscles. This muscle has the same action as the hyoglossus and is sometimes regarded as part of it.

e. The **styloglossus muscle** (extrinsic) arises from the anterior and lateral surfaces of the temporal styloid processes, and from the adjacent part of the stylomandibular ligaments. It passes between the internal and external carotid arteries. As it enters the tongue laterally, it divides into a longitudinal part (which blends with the inferior longitudinal muscle) and an oblique part (which blends with the hyoglossus muscle). The styloglossus muscle acts to draw the tongue upward and backward.

f. The **palatoglossus muscle** (extrinsic) arises from the anterior surface of the soft palate and passes downward in front of the palatine tonsils to insert into the sides of the tongue. It draws the root of the tongue upward to help close the posterior part of the oral cavity when food or fluid is temporarily retained in the mouth (ILLUSTRATION 3-21).

g. The **superior and inferior longitudinal muscles** (intrinsic) run from front to back in the upper and lower parts of the tongue (ILLUSTRATION 3-21). The superior part originates from the median fibrous septum and from the submucous fibrous layer near the epiglottis, and inserts into the anterior edges of the tongue. The inferior portion may have some origin from the hyoid bone. It lies between the genioglossus and hyoglossus muscles, and extends from the root to the apex of the tongue. These muscles act to shorten the length of the tongue, to bend it to either side or to curl the tip upward or downward.

h. Other intrinsic muscles, innervated by the hypoglossal nerve, include the **transverse muscles** (arising from the median fibrous septum and running laterally to insert into the sides of the tongue) and the **vertical muscles** (which connect the upper and lower surfaces of the tongue anteriorly). The transverse muscles narrow the tongue, and the vertical muscles thin its edges.

5. Other muscles attaching to the mandible

a. The **digastric muscle** is biomechanically interesting. It has two origins: a depression on the inner side of the inferior border of the mandible close to the symphysis, and the mastoid notch of the temporal bone (which runs from front to back medially to the base of the mastoid processes). The insertion is onto a tendon located about one-third of the way from the (anterior) mandibular origin to the (posterior) temporal origin. This tendon passes through a loop of connective tissue which is attached to the greater cornua and body of the hyoid bone. This loop sometimes has a synovial sheath for accommodation of movement of the digastric tendon. The tendon passes through the stylohyoideus muscle, which inserts on the hyoid bone near the loop.

The digastric muscle does not form a straight line in its route between the mandible and the temporal bone. It is more inferior where the tendon passes through the loop. This means that the anterior and posterior bellies form two legs of a triangle, the hypotenuse of which would be a straight line connecting the two origins of the muscle (ILLUSTRATION 3-22). Because of this arrangement, when the digastric contracts it raises the hyoid bone as the two legs of the triangle attempt to form a straight line. However, when the hyoid bone is fixed, contraction of the digastric muscle assists the lateral pterygoid muscle in opening the lower jaw. If the mandible and hyoid bone are both fixed, contraction of the digastric muscle will produce internal rotation of the temporal bone, since the temporal origin is posterior and inferior to the bone's axis of rotation.

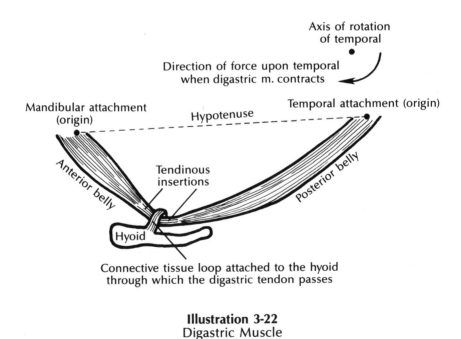

Illustration 3-22
Digastric Muscle

The two bellies of the digastric muscle have separate embryological origins. The anterior belly is derived from the first (mandibular) branchial arch, the posterior belly from the second (hyoid) arch. Accordingly, they have different innervations: the anterior belly is innervated by the mylohyoid branch of the inferior alveolar nerve (part of the mandibular division of the trigeminal nerve), the posterior belly by the digastric branch of the facial nerve (which emerges from the stylomastoid foramen of the temporal bone just anterior to the digastric notch). Deep to the posterior belly, we find the occipital artery which runs between the digastric and the fibers of origin of the levator scapulae muscles. The posterior border of the digastric is just deep to the insertions of the splenius capitis and semispinalis capitis muscles (ILLUSTRATION 3-23).

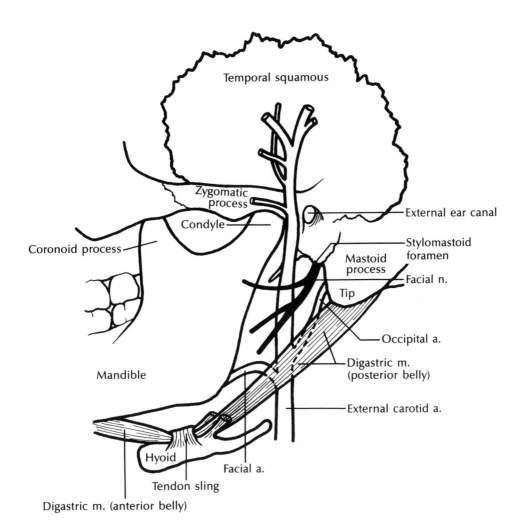

Illustration 3-23
Posterior Belly of the Digastric Muscle

The mid-portion of the posterior belly of the digastric muscle is located behind the angle of the mandible. Deep to this portion of the muscle are the spinal accessory

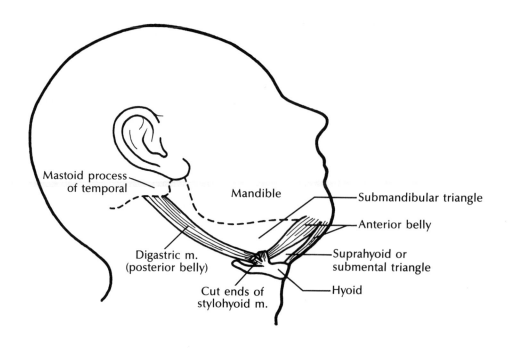

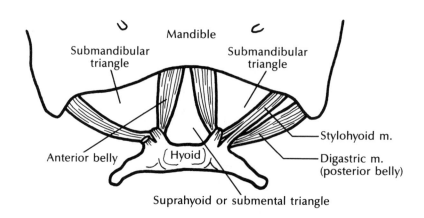

Illustration 3-24
Anterior Belly of the Digastric Muscle

nerve, hypoglossal nerve, internal jugular vein, external carotid artery and deep upper cervical lymph nodes. The internal carotid artery and vagus nerve are located deeper in the neck. Part of the parotid gland is found on the anterior surface of the posterior belly. The submandibular salivary gland is just superficial to the tendon of the digastric. The facial artery runs between the tendon and the mandible before it angles across the mandible to supply the superficial tissues. The anterior belly of the digastric muscle is located on the inferior surface of the mylohyoid muscle. This belly divides the region between the mandible and the hyoid into two triangles on each side of the throat: the submandibular triangle and the suprahyoid (or submental) triangle (ILLUS-TRATION 3-24).

b. The **mylohyoid muscle** (bilateral) forms the muscular floor of the mouth. The line of origin of the muscle (mylohyoid line) on each medial side of the mandible extends from the symphysis menti to the wisdom tooth (third molar). There is an unpaired median raphe of tough connective tissue which extends from the symphysis menti to the midportion of the hyoid body. The mylohyoid inserts onto this raphe and the hyoid. Sometimes the fibers of the two halves of the muscle are continuous across the midline if the raphe is poorly developed. The muscle acts to raise the floor of the mouth and elevate the hyoid bone during swallowing. When the hyoid bone is fixed from below, its contraction assists the lateral pterygoid muscle in lowering the mandible. Innervation is from the mylohyoid branch of the inferior alveolar nerve, part of the mandibular division of the trigeminal system (ILLUSTRATION 3-25).

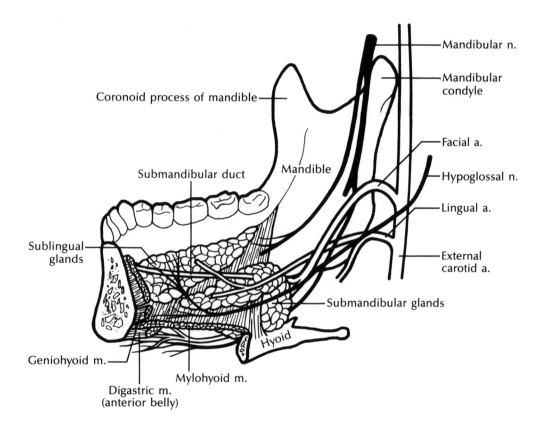

Illustration 3-25
Cross Section of Mylohyoid Muscle

The inferior surface of the mylohyoid muscle is in contact with the anterior digastric muscle, submandibular glands, submental artery, mylohyoid nerve and artery. The superior surface, which contributes to the oral cavity floor, is in contact with the genio-hyoid and other tongue muscles. The submandibular gland wraps around the posterior border of the mylohyoid muscle and is therefore above it in the rear of the mouth. The posterior superior part of the mylohyoid muscle is also in close proximity to the duct of the submandibular gland and sublingual glands, the hypoglossal nerve, lingual nerves and vessels of the tongue.

    c. The **geniohyoid muscle** (bilateral) originates from the inferior mental spine of the symphysis menti and inserts on the anterior hyoid body. The two halves contact each other at the midline. The geniohyoid muscle lies upon the upper surface of the mylohyoid muscle and shares the anatomical relationships described above. Innervation is from a branch of the hypoglossal nerve (most authorities agree that this branch is actually derived from fibers arising from the first cervical root, rather than the hypoglossal system per se) (ILLUSTRATION 3-26). Action of this muscle is the same as that of the mylohyoid.

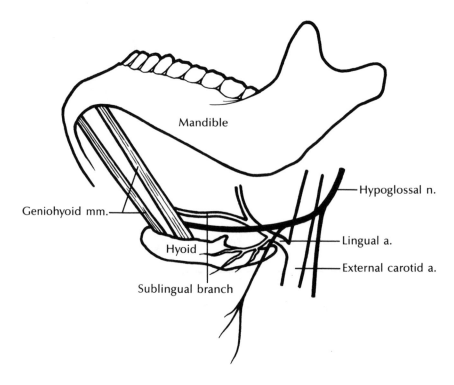

Illustration 3-26
Geniohyoid Muscles

    d. The **platysma** is a broad, thin, superficial, sheet-like muscle with many irregularities on its surface. It arises from the superficial fascia of the pectoral and deltoid muscles, ascends over the clavicles up the anterior neck and inserts onto the mandible and/or the superficial muscles in the area. It acts to depress the mandible and lower lip. Innervation is from the cervical branch of the facial nerve.

IV. TEETH

My friend and colleague, Dr. Richard MacDonald (an osteopathic physician who joined our Institute in July 1987) suggests that we consider the teeth as cranial bones, that we diagnose and treat them as such, and apply the principles and techniques of craniosacral therapy to them. Let us consider the teeth in this context.

The first set of 20 teeth (deciduous) emerge during childhood. They consist of two incisors, one canine and two molars in each quadrant of the mouth. The lower incisors are the first to appear, at approximately six months. Timing is variable, but the full set of deciduous teeth is usually present by the age of 24 months.

The shedding of deciduous teeth and their replacement by permanent teeth begins around six years and is usually completed by age 13, except for the third molars (wisdom teeth). These molars are quite variable in structure, location and time of eruption, which is usually between ages 17 and 25, but can be much later (mine did not appear until my mid-40's). The permanent teeth consist of two incisors, one canine, two premolars and three molars in each quadrant (ILLUSTRATION 3-27).

Each tooth consists of a crown (the part projecting from the gum), root (the articulating part embedded in the alveolus of the maxilla or mandible) and neck (the narrow part connecting the crown and root). The depression in which each root is set is lined with periosteum, which invests the root. At the opening of the alveolus, the periosteal investiture blends with the fibers of the gum. Periodontal disease is the breakdown of this blending.

A thin layer of bone (crusta petrosa) covers each tooth from the neck to the tip of the root. This layer gets thicker as we get older, and develops exostoses. Nerves and blood vessels enter the root through an orifice at the apex. The interior of the tooth, called the pulp canal (from the root to the neck) or pulp chamber (from the neck into the crown), is filled with a highly vascularized and innervated loose connective tissue called "dental pulp." The solid outer layer of the the tooth is made of dentin, a modified type of bone tissue. The hard substance covering the external surface of the crown is enamel. Enamel is composed of tiny hexagonal rods lying parallel to each other, with one end in contact with the underlying dentin and the other forming the external tooth surface (ILLUSTRATION 3-28).

The junction of each tooth root with its bone constitutes a gomphosis type of fibrous joint (SECTION II.B.1), and slight movement is possible. As with any joint, excessive and/or repeated stress upon one component (the tooth in this case) may cause joint degeneration, leading to looseness or pain in the tooth. Rehabilitation of this joint and the periosteum may be aided by gentle manipulation of the teeth or jaw so that physiological motion is enhanced. V-spread techniques are also appropriate (SECTION VII).

V. BIOMECHANICS

In opening the mouth, we move the mandible (lower jaw) away from the maxilla (upper jaw). For protection of the tissues on the side of the head near the external ear canal, the axis of rotation of the mandible is low on the ramus or angle, 4-6cm below the articulating condyle. Thus, the condyle must move forward in order for the mouth to open. Since the temporal bone is relatively fixed, this means the condyle

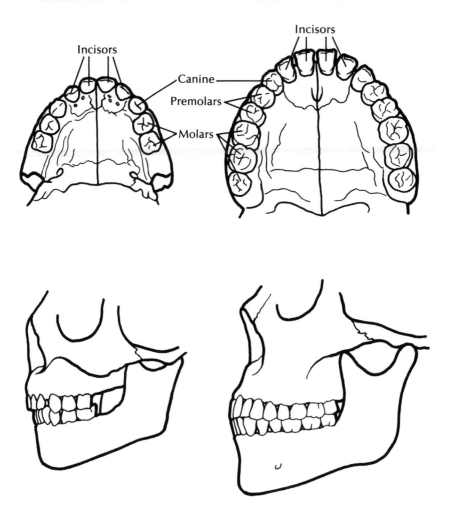

1 — DECIDUOUS TEETH   2 — PERMANENT TEETH

Illustration 3-27
Distribution of Deciduous and Permanent Teeth

must glide forward (up to 2cm in some cases) in relation to the temporal. For this purpose, a unique joint surface is provided by the temporal, resembling an "S" lying on its side with the convexity upward posteriorly (the fossa) and downward anteriorly (the articular eminence) (SECTION II.C.1).

When the mouth is opened, the condyle travels forward, down the anterior slope of the fossa which is also the posterior slope of the articular eminence. As the angle of opening increases, the condyle passes over the downward aimed peak of the eminence and moves along the upward slanting anterior slope (ILLUSTRATION 3-29). If you place your fingers over the condyles and open your mouth widely, you can detect the movement described.

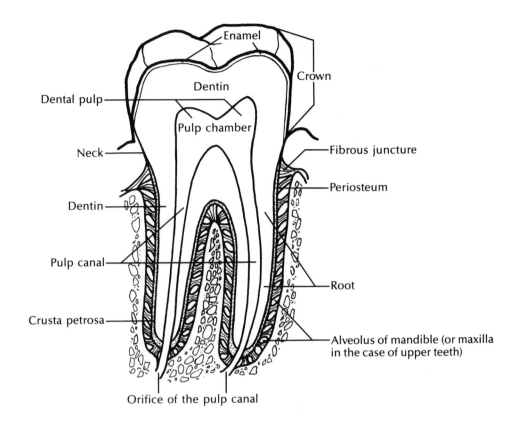

Illustration 3-28
Anatomy of a Tooth

The interarticular disc (SECTION II.C.3) between the articulating bones is attached to the lateral and medial poles of the condyle by the collateral ligaments. It is allowed to move about the cylindrically shaped superior surface of the condyle on a transverse axis which passes through the two poles; it acts much as a bearing in a crank shaft or a piston pin, and protects the two joint surfaces. It is actually the disc-condyle complex which articulates with the temporal in order to accommodate movements of the mandible in relation to the maxilla (ILLUSTRATION 3-30).

What keeps the disc interposed between the condyle and the temporal surface during jaw movement? There are three major factors. First, the superior portion of the lateral pterygoid muscle, by its contraction, moves the disc forward in relation to the condyle. Second, the retrodiscal tissue (SECTION II.D) acts as an elastic resistance and memory tissue which counter-balances the action of the superior lateral pterygoid on the disc. Third, the disc is thicker posteriorly and therefore resists to some extent the forward movement encouraged by the superior lateral pterygoid as the condyle is compressed against the temporal joint surface (ILLUSTRATION 3-31). In fact, compression of the two bony surfaces by the mandibular sling muscles tends to "squirt" the disc backward.

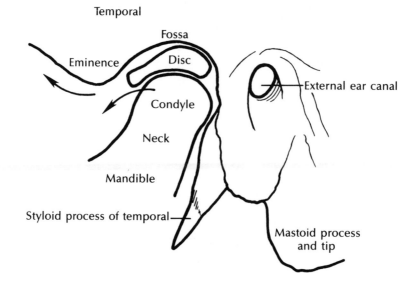

Illustration 3-29
Movement of the Mandibular Condyle
When the Mouth is Opened

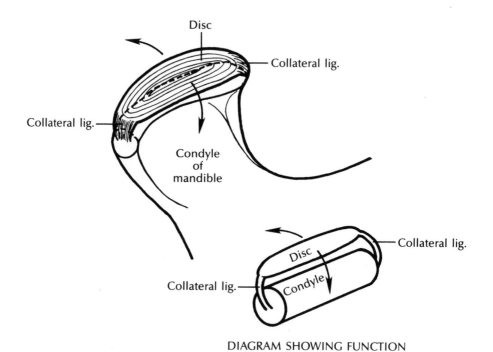

DIAGRAM SHOWING FUNCTION

Illustration 3-30
Disc-Condyle Complex

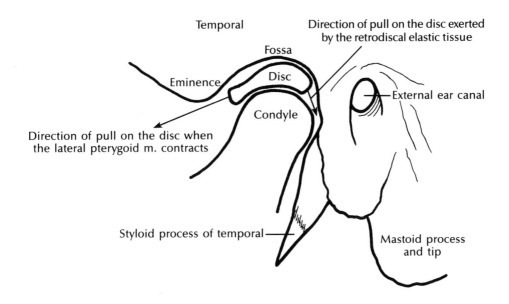

Illustration 3-31
Biomechanics of the Interarticular Disc

Elevation of the mandible is produced by contraction of the temporalis, masseter and medial pterygoid muscles. Depression of the mandible is produced primarily by the inferior part of the lateral pterygoids, and secondarily by the mylohyoid, digastric and geniohyoid muscles, assuming the hyoid bone is fixed from below. Anterior protrusion of the jaw is produced by contraction of the lateral pterygoid muscles with simultaneous contraction of the jaw closure muscles, jaw retraction by contraction of the posterior fibers of the temporalis muscle.

The collateral ligaments of the interarticular disc hold it in its proper relationship to the condyle. The capsule acts as a "boot" for the joint, offering attachment for the retrodiscal tissue, which is partially elastic and partially ligamentous. The temporomandibular and sphenomandibular ligaments dictate the mandible's axis of rotation and prevent posterior and inferior jaw dislocation. The stylomandibular ligament connects the posterior angle of the mandible with the temporal; it prevents inferior dislocation of the joint and stabilizes the cervical fascia.

How do the teeth relate to temporomandibular joint function? At rest the upper and lower teeth are separated; when the jaw is forcibly closed, they come into contact. The surfaces of the teeth are not horizontally flush. As pressure increases, they begin to mesh much like the teeth of two saw blades being forced together (ILLUSTRATION 3-32).

As the mandible is elevated more forcibly, the position of maximal intercuspation (teeth compressed together) is reached. If the condyle has not been forced to move, and has not been excessively compressed into the temporomandibular joint complex, there is no harm done. However, if the condyle is forced to change position in relation to the temporal joint surface, friction and eventual joint deterioration will result. Alternatively, if the molars lack proper height, forcible closure of the mandible may

1 — TEETH NOT TOUCHING

2 — TEETH OCCLUDE PROPERLY
WHEN MOUTH CLOSES

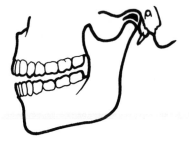 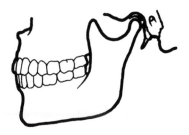

Illustration 3-32-A
Proper Occlusion of Teeth with No Ill-Effects
on Temporomandibular Joint

1 — TEETH IMPROPERLY OCCLUDED
(EXAGGERATED)

2 — FULL CLOSURE FORCES
CONDYLE POSTERIORLY

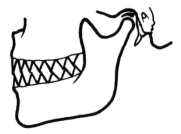 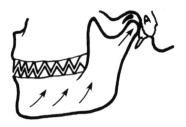

Illustration 3-32-B
Improper Occlusion of Teeth with Impaction
of Temporomandibular Joint

excessively impact the condyle into the joint, again resulting in eventual joint damage (ILLUSTRATION 3-33).

As in any joint, proper function of the temporomandibular joint depends on sensory information from the joint components and related structures (i.e., muscles, teeth and periodontal receptors). Distortion of sensory input concerning degree of joint compression may lead to overcompression and eventual TMJ syndrome. For example, biting an object too hard with the incisors causes compression of the temporomandibular joint because the molars are not acting to prevent overcompression (ILLUSTRATION 3-34). Sensory input from temporomandibular joint-associated structures is necessary to prevent damage in this situation. Certainly, the temporalis, masseter and medial pterygoid muscles have sufficient power to severely damage the inter-

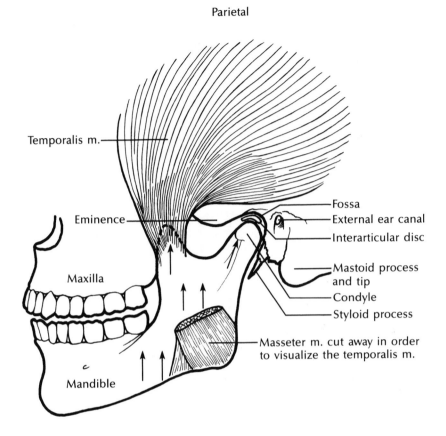

Parietal

Temporalis m.—

Eminence—

Maxilla

Mandible

Fossa
External ear canal
Interarticular disc
Mastoid process and tip
Condyle
Styloid process
Masseter m. cut away in order to visualize the temporalis m.

Illustration 3-33
Mechanics of TMJ Compression

articular disc and other joint structures were it not for this type of sensory input. Similarly, distortion of sensory input from teeth may be involved in bruxism (teeth grinding).

VI. TMJ SYNDROME

A. Introduction

Primary symptoms related to what is called "TMJ syndrome" are: painful chewing; inability to either fully or partially open or close the mouth; noise when chewing or opening or closing the mouth (clicking, popping, crepitus); abnormal sensations associated with jaw movement; zigzag movements associated with jaw movement; malocclusion; ear symptoms such as pressure, tinnitus or pain; referred pain to face, head or neck. There are many possible causes for these symptoms. Some of them relate to the temporomandibular joint and some do not. I cannot emphasize enough that

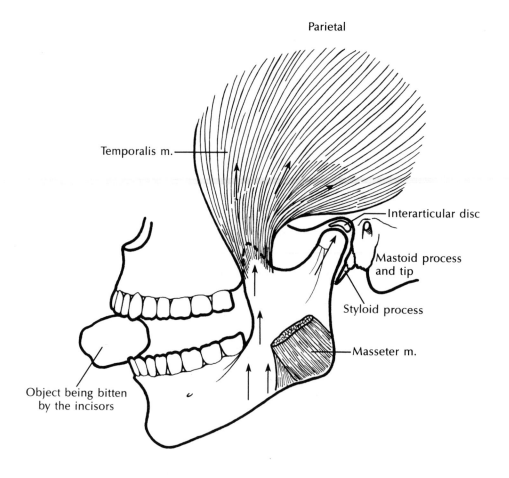

Illustration 3-34
Effect of Incisor Biting Upon the TMJ

whole body diagnosis is essential in order to determine whether the apparent temporomandibular joint problem is one of cause or effect. Some possible causes are listed below. Of course, there may be more than one cause for TMJ syndrome in a particular patient.

B. Causes

1. Chronic malocclusion creates friction in the joint each time the jaw is forcibly closed. The end of closure causes a last minute repositioning of the joint components in order to accommodate the demands of the teeth as they interface maximally. You can see this by asking the patient to just barely touch the teeth together and then clench tight. If this problem is present, you will see the upper and lower teeth shift in relationship to each other as the jaws are tightly clenched. You may also feel the condyles move in relation to the temporal bones at this moment.

2. Loss of vertical height in the molars results when these teeth are absent, worn down or ground down by a dentist. In this situation, clenching of the teeth will produce an obvious compression of one or both temporomandibular joints. When you use the craniosacral temporomandibular joint decompression techniques, you can feel the condyle come out of the temporal fossa; the compression reoccurs when the teeth are clenched again.

I am reminded of a woman in her early 20's whom I treated while I was at Michigan State University. She was suffering from inability to open her mouth more than 2cm, along with temporomandibular joint pain and frequent severe head and neck pain. In an attempt to improve her occlusion, a dentist had ground down her molars several months earlier. This resulted in abnormal compression of the temporomandibular joint, with a secondary tendency to internal rotation of the temporal bones. I used temporomandibular joint decompression techniques (UPLEDGER 1983:199-202 and APPENDIX G), which resulted in a significant improvement in all symptoms. However, following treatment, the stature of the molars was insufficient to maintain the positive effect. The patient used the self-help techniques described in my first book to maintain the decompression until another dentist was able to restore satisfactory vertical stature to the molars.

3. The **articular eminence** of the temporal bone may have very steep sides, making it difficult for the condyle-disc complex to ascend or descend. This condition is palpable as extreme inferior and superior excursion of the condyle upon opening or closing; an X-ray will confirm the diagnosis. I have seen this condition only rarely, but am reminded of a female teenage patient whose mouth was locked wide open. X-rays revealed very steep slopes to the articular eminences, particularly anteriorly. The condyles had traveled down the posterior slopes, past the apices of the eminences and gone up the anterior slope. At this point, pain caused muscle contraction which would not allow the condyles to come back over the apices without assistance. That assistance came in the form of some diazepam (Valium) for muscle relaxation and calming effect, followed by gentle but firm assisting traction to help the condyles move inferiorly and posteriorly over the apices. The patient was advised not to open her mouth so wide in the future. I do not know of any other effective approach in such a case.

4. There may be damage to one or both of the temporomandibular joints due to **trauma.** Since this is a gliding joint, the surface must be smooth even though it is curved. Interruption in the smoothness of the normal gliding movement is palpable as "hitch" in the movement, and/or crepitus. X-ray, and history of trauma, may be needed to confirm this diagnosis.

5. Nervous habits and/or tics may contribute to temporomandibular joint abuse and eventual dysfunction. Among these are bruxism, chronic jaw clenching, chronic chewing on one side, and a variety of other idiosyncrasies.

6. The **interarticular disc** may escape (usually forward) from between the condyle and the temporal joint surface. Since the disc is wider posteriorly, it may be difficult to get it back between the two bony surfaces. Gentle decompression may do the job. If the disc remains displaced, the condyle begins to compress and abuse the retrodiscal tissue, causing it to lose its elasticity, which in turn makes the return of the disc to its normal position when the lateral pterygoid muscle relaxes less probable. Causes of such anterior displacement include chronic hypertonus of the lateral pterygoid muscle, nutritional deficiencies or trauma (acute or chronic) affecting the retrodiscal tissue and its elasticity.

7. Spasms of the muscles of mastication may result from strain, trauma or inflammation. The involved muscle can usually be localized by palpation and motion testing of the mandible.

8. Inflammation of the joint capsule or associated ligaments can be localized by palpation and arcing techniques (UPLEDGER 1983, CHAPTER 14), further described in chapter 4 below.

9. Joint problems such as arthritis and ankylosis can occur in the temporomandibular joint. In my experience, the temporomandibular joint is comparatively resilient and these conditions are quite rare; they are usually reversible by craniosacral techniques when they do occur.

10. The most frequent offenders in TMJ syndrome are the **temporal bones.** They are frequently out of synchrony, i.e., one externally rotated, the other in internal rotation. The external end of the axis of rotation of the temporal is 1-2cm posterior to the resting position of the condyle in the temporal fossa. The angulation of the axis (which runs approximately through the external auditory meatus) is antero-medial on a roughly horizontal plane. Thus, when the temporal bone is restricted in external rotation, the fossa is displaced downward slightly (or upward in the case of internal rotation), which in turn moves the condyle inferiorly (or superiorly) on the side of the affected temporal bone. When chronic, this situation may result in temporomandibular joint dysfunction which is clearly an effect rather than a cause.

When you discover temporal bone dysfunction, you must determine its cause. Such dysfunction may be (1) primary; (2) the result of something as close at hand as a cervical problem via the sternocleidomastoid, or an occipital problem; or (3) the result of something as distant as a sacral dysfunction which transmits its restriction up to the temporal bone via the dural tube to the upper cervicals and the occiput, or directly through the transverse membrane system (tentorium cerebelli). Of course, such a sacral problem could be coming from almost anywhere below the respiratory diaphragm. The body must be considered as an integrated whole when the practitioner attempts to determine the underlying reasons for temporomandibular joint problems which may appear localized.

I once treated a 58-year-old woman referred by a dentist. She was under care for temporomandibular joint dysfunction for over a year, with splints and devices to balance and correct the bite, without success. She suffered from a chronically unlevel sacral base (right side low) and occiput. The occipital problem created dysfunction of the cranial base with bilateral temporal bone dysfunction, and secondary temporomandibular joint problem. Because the sphenoid was compensating for the occipital unlevelling, the pterygoid processes produced a torsional dysfunction of the hard palate which the dentist was trying to correct. The oral work was not clinically effective until the sacral base and occipital unlevellings were corrected, after which the temporomandibular joint problem improved rapidly and the oral devices became unnecessary.

11. TMJ syndrome may also arise from the relation of the **hard palate** to the mandible below and the sphenoid above. Any rotational dysfunction of the maxilla will create a malocclusion. Many such malocclusions are corrected in the course of craniosacral therapy; by the time the temporal bones are balanced, the hard palate has been released and balanced, and the temporomandibular joints have been decompressed. Look to the maxilla when there is last second realignment of the teeth upon power clenching. You cannot correct the maxilla without attending to the vomer, palatines and sphenoid; we see again the importance of whole body diagnosis.

A frequent cause of maxillary dysfunction is the leverage applied during the extraction of a molar (especially a wisdom tooth). I experienced this phenomenon several years ago when my upper right wisdom tooth was extracted. My bite changed, my right temporomandibular joint became uncomfortable and I began having right sided midcervical discomfort as well as headache (to which I have seldom been victim). Fortunately I understood the problem, evaluated my own hard palate and found the right maxillary restricted in internal rotation. I corrected this dysfunction and the whole "syndrome" disappeared immediately.

C. Disc problems

The dental profession has classified interarticular disc problems into four classes (I-IV). Class I is assigned when the mandible slides to one side or the other, or forward or backward, when the teeth are forcibly clenched. Class II includes painless clicks upon opening the jaw after maximum clenching. Class III involves pain in the temporomandibular joint, restricted movement and a sense of malocclusion (more probably due to joint surface damage and disc-condyle complex dysfunction, in my opinion). Class IV involves subluxation due to severe disc-condyle complex failure: the disc has probably escaped backward and the condyle is forward, the jaw is stuck open and there is considerable pain.

Incidentally, it is my belief that classification schemes such as this one frequently interfere with the diagnostic effort. Often, a patient is classified, and then given the treatment assigned to that classification. It matters little whether or not his condition improves; what matters is that he is receiving the "proper" treatment. In fact, diagnosis must be continually pursued. It is better to discover a new diagnosis on each visit than to obstinately try to force the patient to fit your original diagnosis and be "correct" on paper even as the condition worsens or remains unchanged.

D. Diagnosis

The craniosacral diagnosis of temporomandibular joint dysfunction is straightforward. Use the compression-decompression technique (UPLEDGER 1983, CHAPTER 12). If there is an imbalance in either phase of the technique, you know that there is a dysfunction of the temporomandibular joint. If one side "compresses" more easily than the other, the side which compresses less is already compressed. As the mandible is tractioned in an inferior direction, it will move toward the side of the "stuck" or chronically compressed temporomandibular joint. Muscle tensions should be observed for imbalance as you decompress. The direction which the mandible follows during the technique will clearly indicate the diagnosis.

VII. CRANIOSACRAL TREATMENT OF TEMPOROMANDIBULAR JOINT DYSFUNCTION

Craniosacral treatment of the TMJ syndrome is based on whole person diagnosis. First, you acknowledge the presence of the symptoms in the temporomandibular joint or masticatory system. Next, you must search for the cause.

Begin with whole body diagnosis, using the techniques of arcing, fascial glide and evaluation of craniosacral motion for symmetry and quality (UPLEDGER 1983, CHAPTER 14), further described in chapter 4 below. Find the restrictions in the body of the patient. By palpation, evaluate temporomandibular joint and mandibular balance (UPLEDGER 1983, CHAPTER 12). Then treat the body restrictions you have found (using whatever techniques seem appropriate) and reevaluate the effects of that treatment.

Evaluate the total craniosacral system from sacrum to occiput and the intracranial membrane system, the vertical falxes and the horizontal tentorium cerebelli (UPLEDGER 1983, CHAPTER 6). Correct what you find and reevaluate temporomandibular joint and mandibular balance. This process will give you more information about causes. Improvement of temporomandibular joint function by the correction of external, distant restrictions reflects that the temporomandibular joint symptoms are effect, not cause. In fact, you should realize at this point that the cause probably lies outside the masticatory system.

As you work, pay special attention to the temporal bones, their mobility and their relationship to the horizontal membrane system and sutures. Be sure that temporal restriction is not coming from the extrinsic muscles which are attached to the bone (sternocleidomastoid, temporalis, digastric, longissimus capitis, splenius capitis, masseter and stylohyoideus). Of these muscles, the sternocleidomastoid, temporalis and masseter are easily palpable, and their tonicity easily evaluated. Hypertonicity of the sternocleidomastoid is palpable along the lateral part of the upper neck and the anterior part of the lower throat. The muscle runs diagonally between the mastoid process and the sternoclavicular joint. It is innervated by the spinal accessory nerve and branches of C2 and C3. Abnormal hypertonus or contracture of this muscle tends to pull the mastoid process downward and forward. Since the temporal bone's axis of rotation is anterior to and slightly above the muscle attachment, this causes the temporal bone to be resistant to external rotation (i.e., flexion of the craniosacral system). It may, in fact, lock the temporal bone in internal rotation (ILLUSTRATION 3-35).

The bodies of C2 and C3 are attached to the dural tube within the vertebral canal. This means that a dural tube problem from as far away as the sacrum can easily create dysfunction of these vertebrae, a condition which may contribute, via the related nerve roots, to abnormal tonus of the sternocleidomastoid. This in turn causes temporal bone dysfunction, as well as dysfunction of the occipitomastoid suture which the muscle attachment crosses. Temporal bone and sutural dysfunction may then create problems at the jugular foramen (CHAPTER 1, SECTION IX). The spinal accessory nerve exits through

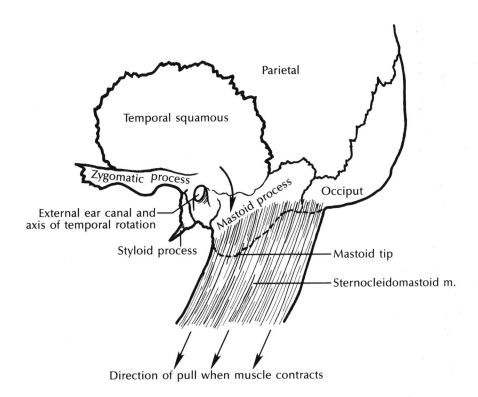

Illustration 3-35
Effect of the Sternocleidomastoid Muscle
on the Temporal

this foramen, as do the glossopharyngeal nerve, vagus nerve and jugular vein (ILLUS-TRATION 3-36). Compression of the foramen can compress and hypersensitize the accessory nerve, which in turn increases the hypertonicity of the sternocleidomastoid, further compressing the nerve in a vicious circle.

The glossopharyngeal nerve carries sensory taste information from the posterior third of the tongue (CHAPTER 1, SECTION VII), responding mostly to bitter or salty substances. Loss of this sense is not usually a cause for complaint by a patient. In fact, the patient may tell you that food is tasting better.

On the other hand, the vagus nerve (CHAPTER 1, SECTION VIII), when hypersensitized by compression at the jugular foramen, can produce a variety of undesirable symptoms. These include light-headedness, syncopal (fainting) episodes, heart racing or irregularity, air-hunger (inability to ''catch a good breath''), excessive stomach acid (heartburn), pyloric dysfunction (interfering with passage of digested food into the small intestine) and large intestine dysfunction (manifested as irregularity).

Pressure on the jugular vein at the jugular foramen results in what I call ''fluid congestion head,'' i.e., a slight increase in fluid back pressure, causing the fluid volume and pressure within the cranial vault to increase. This results in headache (''feels like my head wants to explode''; ''lots of pressure behind my eyes,'' etc.); the inability

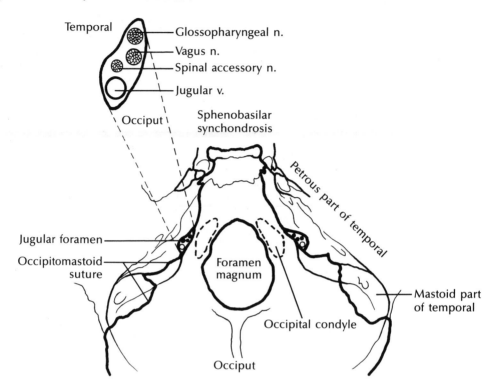

ENLARGED INSET VIEW
OF JUGULAR FORAMEN

Temporal — Glossopharyngeal n.
— Vagus n.
— Spinal accessory n.
— Jugular v.

Occiput — Sphenobasilar synchondrosis

Petrous part of temporal

Jugular foramen
Occipitomastoid suture

Foramen magnum

Mastoid part of temporal

Occipital condyle

Occiput

Illustration 3-36
Jugular Foramen

to concentrate, organize one's thoughts or remember things; and possibly some pituitary dysfunction.

Techniques to release the jugular foramen involve the mobilization of the occiput and temporal bone in relation to each other. I seldom use a single technique, but instead visualize the functional anatomy and start moving the two bones in the easiest and most anatomically logical way possible. That is, find the motion that is present and exaggerate that motion until the whole unit frees up. I begin by releasing the occipital cranial base (UPLEDGER 1983, CHAPTER 5). Be sure the thoracic inlet has been freed before you release the occipital cranial base. During the process of base release, you will effectively be relaxing the longissimus capitis and splenius capitis muscles, both of which attach to the posterior mastoid process. The longissimus capitis generally originates from the articular processes of vertebrae C4 through T5 inclusive. It lies deep to the splenius capitis, which originates from the lower half of the nuchal ligament and from the spinous processes of vertebrae C7 to T4. Both of these muscles act to extend the head backward. In so doing, they encourage the temporal bones to rotate internally (extension of the craniosacral system) and resist external rotation. Problems in the middle and lower cervical spine are often referred to the temporal bones via these muscles, both of which are innervated by the middle and lower cervical nerve roots. You may be tempted to blame neck pain and middle-lower cervical somatic dysfunction on temporomandibular joint problems, rather than vice versa. Remember that joints are usually "slaves" to soft tissue rather than the other way around.

After releasing the occipital base, you need to stabilize the occiput while you move the temporal bone. Simply place one hand under the occiput as though you were performing the vault hold with one thumb over the sphenoid wing, and do the temporal ear pull technique with the other hand. After the temporal has released laterally, do the circumferential temporal bone technique, putting the bone through its internal-external rotation range of motion several times in order to free it from the occiput, as you continue to stabilize the latter bone with your other hand. These techniques, followed by a functional "unwinding" of the temporal if it seems desirable, will free up the jugular foramen.

Hypertonus of the temporalis or masseter muscles (both of which are innervated by the trigeminal system) is readily palpable just under the skin. Compression-decompression of the temporomandibular joint with mandibular balancing will frequently release these contractions. Often the cause of such hypertonus is chronic anger or tension. These possibilities must be explored and alleviated in order to obtain free mobility of the temporal bone. The temporalis muscle connects the squamous portion of the temporal bone to the coronoid process of the mandible, while the masseter connects the zygomatic arch to the ramus and angle of the mandible. Both are gently released and balanced during the decompression phase of the technique. Position-and-hold (also known as counterstrain) techniques can also be useful for hypertonus of these muscles (JONES 1981).

The posterior digastric muscle connects the temporal bone (just medial to the base of the mastoid process) to the hyoid bone; the stylohyoid muscle connects the styloid process of the temporal bone to the hyoid bone. Both muscles are innervated by branches of the facial nerve system. With the hyoid bone fixed, contraction of either or both muscles will internally rotate the temporal bone, i.e., cause extension of the craniosacral system. Hyoid palpation will reveal the condition of the muscles. Gently place your hands over the temporal bones as though you are doing the temporomandibular joint decompression technique. Let your fingertips move down to the hyoid bone and move it slowly and gently in an inferior direction. See if this causes an uneven effect upon the temporal bones. Gently balance the hyoid bone while holding the temporal bones still with the palms of your hands. This will release the muscles. Release of the temporal bones and the tentorium cerebelli will do a lot to decompress any pressure on the facial nerve as it travels within the cranial vault and through the osseous canals within the temporal bone.

There are two other muscles which attach to the temporal bone (styloglossus and auricular posterior), but to my knowledge they are not capable of restricting temporal bone motion.

Another area which must be thoroughly evaluated and treated when dealing with potential TMJ syndrome is the hard palate (maxilla, palatines, vomer) (UPLEDGER 1983, CHAPTER 12). The dental occlusion will change significantly when there is correction of a hard palate problem, and therefore occlusal work by a dental specialist before the hard palate and temporal bones are thoroughly mobilized is not recommended.

After you have decompressed the hard palate in an anterior direction, it is necessary that you move the mandible (lower jaw) forward into alignment with the maxillae.

To do this, simply repeat the decompression phase of the technique you used for temporomandibular joint release and mandibular balancing prior to the hard palate work. At the end of the decompression technique, encourage the mandible to move forward so that the upper and lower teeth may better occlude when the mouth is closed. Do not force the mandible to move anteriorly, but do offer it the opportunity, and encourage it to take advantage of that opportunity, in a very gentle manner.

The concept of treating teeth as cranial bones has been mentioned (SECTION IV). My clinical observations suggest that the direction of energy (V-spread) technique through a tooth, performed regularly, may revitalize the pulp of the tooth and obviate the need for extraction or root canal work. Furthermore, gentle mobilization of the teeth in their sockets will enhance their ability to adapt to occlusal changes and thus reduce the number of times that orthodontic correction of malocclusion is necessary. Given the chance, the teeth may adjust to bite changes; craniosacral therapy simply enhances their adaptability. Cooperative patients should be taught to work with their own teeth in this way.

The techniques for teeth require some creative ingenuity. I think that it is best to direct the energy longitudinally through the tooth. In the lower jaw, place the sending finger under the mandible and the receiving fingers on either side of the biting surface of the tooth. For upper teeth, send from the top of the head through the tooth with the receiving fingers on each side of its biting surface. My best results have come from sending the energy from the root to the crown. Abscesses will respond to transversely directed energy. If in doubt, do it both vertically and transversely. You can't hurt anything, and you may help.

To help the teeth adjust to an occlusal problem, place your fingertip on the biting surface of the tooth and help it "unwind." Let your fingers go where they want to; trust them. I cannot be definite in terms of technique description here because each case is different and requires creative improvisation. Let your intuition tell you how to treat each tooth. Changes resulting from the "unwinding" of a tooth require time and repeated treatments. It doesn't always work, but when it does, it can eliminate the need for extensive dental work.

I am often asked about splints. I believe the purpose of the dental splint should be to prevent the impaction of the condyle into the temporomandibular joint when there has been loss of the vertical height of the molars. When the "splinters" try to go further with their appliances, they begin to interfere with the natural adaptive and remodeling ability of the joint tissues. The temporomandibular joint is one of the most, if not the most, resilient joints in the body. Nurture it, take the stress off it and let it heal in its own way. The splint should do no more than reduce the pressure on the joint. There is no reason for the splint to be applied to the upper teeth. It should only be placed on the mandible and must not interfere with the amplitude and vitality of craniosacral system motion. When a splint is applied, you should be able to monitor craniosacral rhythm. If the pressure of the splint restricts the freedom of craniosacral motion in any way, it is not properly fitted. An upper splint stands a much better chance of interfering with maxillary motion in terms of internal and external rotation. A lower splint is much more forgiving, but it can also interfere with craniosacral motion if it presses too hard laterally on the teeth. I have seen splints that totally shut down craniosacral rhythm; I believe this is probably a response to the material used in construction of the splint.

I use a great deal of temporomandibular joint compression-decompression technique (UPLEDGER 1983, CHAPTER 12) very successfully for patients whose temporomandibular joint problems persist after all the aforementioned problems have been resolved. Training of patients in the use of self-help techniques for temporomandibular joint decompression has also been very effective. We advise the use of the technique upon arising, after each meal, and at bed time. Thus, the joint is decompressed five times a day: after the possible stress of a dream-filled night, after chewing and possibly compressing the joint and after the long day to alleviate further stress-induced compression. We are trying to undo the effect of temporomandibular joint compression due to clenching of the teeth, whether resulting from chewing or emotional tension. One of the self-help techniques is described in my first book (UPLEDGER 1983, APPENDIX G). Since that writing, we have found that it is also effective and much more convenient to simply teach the patient to manually decompress the temporomandibular joints directly without the aid of the fulcrums.

This technique was shown to us by one of the dentists who took our intermediate workshop. The patient should: (1) gently place his hands so that the fingers go up the mandibular rami, and the angles of the mandible are in the palms of the hands; (2) very easily and gently, so as not to stimulate muscular resistance, apply traction down the length of the ramus to decompress the joints; (3) hold the traction until he can sense the decompression of both joints. This technique requires a little more sensitivity and instruction for the patient, but once learned, compliance is generally higher because there are no fulcra to put in the mouth, and the technique can be performed less conspicuously.

We also use biofeedback, relaxation techniques and psychotherapy to round out the treatment of what appears to be simple "TMJ syndrome."

VIII. TEMPOROMANDIBULAR JOINT: SUMMARY

The craniosacral therapist must understand the temporomandibular joint, how it works, what it does and how its function is affected by other body parts. Causal factors arising from distant body regions should be considered and investigated. The craniosacral system must be reasonably clear of restrictions and imbalances. The hard palate must be mobile and balanced. When all of this is done, we can begin to appraise just how much of the problem is related to primary dysfunction of the masticatory system and/or the temporomandibular joint. It is clear that, in the future, the significance of the craniosacral system in the diagnosis and treatment of "TMJ syndrome" will be more fully appreciated by the dental profession. Ideally, a competent craniosacral therapist should work in collaboration with the dentist on patients with temporomandibular joint problems.

4.

CLINICAL TECHNIQUES

CHAPTER 4

I. INTRODUCTION

This chapter is at once the most challenging and the most enjoyable for me to write. It is the most challenging because I have little solid scientific evidence, tried and tested, behind which I can hide; almost all the material presented here consists of hypotheses derived from years of clinical observation. It is the most enjoyable because the creative part of me is bursting at the seams, wanting to let my readers in on the sometimes astounding things I have observed as I follow the trail deeper into the mysteries of the craniosacral system and its relevance to the overall health and well-being of the patient.

I realize that some of the subjects discussed here were covered in my first book (UPLEDGER 1983). Five years and many clinical experiences have passed since I wrote that book, with its early descriptions of whole body diagnosis and somatoemotional release and recall. At first, I considered attempting to integrate that material into the present chapter. However, so much has been changed and added that I think it is better to start fresh. If you discover contradictions, please be tolerant. The art of craniosacral therapy changes daily, which is what makes it so exciting. It is also slightly frustrating to know that soon after this book goes to press, I will wish that I could revise it. However, even if the underlying concepts undergo modification, the techniques described here will still be useful. Feel free to modify the techniques in light of your own observations.

A glossary, with definitions and discussions of selected terms and concepts, appears at the back of this book. Please refer to it as necessary. This chapter will assume familiarity with those terms, as well as with the content of my first book.

II. FINDING AND TREATING DISEASE PROCESSES

I will begin (SECTIONS II.A-D) by presenting some concepts which are integral to the remainder of this chapter, and which may be new to some of my readers.

A. Energy cysts

This concept developed over a period of several months at the Michigan State University College of Osteopathic Medicine as I worked with Drs. Zvi Karni (biophysics, biological engineering) and Ernest Retzlaff (neurophysiology). We benefitted from discussions with Drs. Fred Becker (anatomy), Jon Kabara (biochemistry), David McConnell (psychology, biochemistry) and Irwin M. Korr (physiology). The term "energy cyst" was first coined by Elmer Green, Director of the Menninger Foundation in Topeka, Kansas, while he was attending one of my seminar/workshops.

The energy cyst is a construct of our imagination which may have objective reality. We believe that it manifests as an obstruction to the efficient conduction of electricity through the body tissues (primarily fasciae) where it resides, acts as an irritant contributing to the development of the facilitated segment (SECTION II.B), and as a localized irritable focus. As such, it sends out the interference waves which we palpate by arcing techniques (SECTION II.C). In terms of acupuncture theory, we believe that it obstructs the flow of "chi" along the meridians of acupuncture (SEE GLOSSARY). By palpation, one can find the obstruction in the meridian which passes through the energy cyst.

The energy cyst is a localized area of increased entropy, which the host's body has "walled off." Entropy is described by the second law of thermodynamics, which says that all energy moves from the orderly to the disorderly. It takes organizational energy to reverse this natural tendency. When we speak of increased entropy in a human body, we mean an area in which the energy is less orderly or less organized than it is in nearby areas.

The cyst is hotter, more energetic, less organized and less functional than surrounding tissues. It can result from physical trauma, pathogenic invasion, physiological dysfunction, mental and/or emotional problems and (possibly) spiritual problems as well. Sometimes malfunctioning chakras (SEE GLOSSARY) are hosts to energy cysts; release of the cyst is followed by a palpable return of normal chakram function.

The idea of a traumatic origin is easiest to entertain. A blow to the point of the shoulder by a hammer, or the impact on the sacrococcygeal complex during an unexpected fall, puts a force into the recipient's body. What happens to this force? How can the body deal with it? The force represents "excess" energy which the body first tries to dissipate as heat. If successful, the energy leaves the body, normal healing follows and there is no after-effect. If the energy cannot be dissipated as heat, the body (according to our theory) concentrates and localizes the energy, and somehow encapsulates it as an energy cyst, or focus of increased entropy. The body adapts somewhat to the presence of the energy cyst, but in the process ideal function is compromised. Facilitated segments form, fascial mobility is compromised, interference waves are produced, normal electrical conductivity of involved body tissues is reduced and the flow of energy along involved acupuncture meridians is obstructed. All of this compromise saps body energy and creates pain and dysfunction.

We believe that three factors are crucial in determining whether the body is able to dissipate the traumatic energy. First, the quantity of energy may overpower the body's ability to dissipate it. Second, previous injuries to the same body region may have compromised its ability to dissipate the energy. And third, certain emotional states (severe anger, fear, guilt or other negative emotions) paralyze the body's ability to dissipate the energy.

A powerful determining factor in the formation of energy cysts is the emotional status of the subject at the time of injury. If strong negative feelings are dominant at that time, the injury forces will probably be retained and an energy cyst formed. We have seen over and over again that those people who retain the effects of injuries are the ones who harbor anger, resentment, fear, etc., in relation to the accident. Once these negative emotions are discovered and released, the energy cyst/somatic dysfunction and its attendant symptoms are free to leave the subject's body.

Two other factors must be mentioned here: the location of the cyst and the time course of energy dissipation. The location of the cyst depends upon how deeply the traumatic energy penetrates the recipient's body. This in turn depends upon the magnitude of the force and the density of the tissue involved; e.g., a force will penetrate bone less effectively than it will the soft tissue of the abdomen. By "time course" I mean that dissipation of the energy must begin almost immediately after it is absorbed. It may continue for several hours or even days. My impression is that the body makes an "all or none" decision (dissipation vs. localization) at the time of the injury or within the first few minutes thereafter. After this choice is made, the process of either dissipation or localization will continue until completion.

It is not too difficult to imagine that a group of pathogenic invaders can also be walled off as an energy cyst even after the pathogens have been destroyed. The energy of inflammation can be analogized to the traumatic force energy. Likewise, the inflammation secondary to a physiologic dysfunction such as a myocardial infarction or a malignant growth might well be responsible for the formation of an energy cyst under a process, and subject to modifying factors, similar to those described for external trauma.

The concept becomes more difficult to discuss when we move into the realms of mind, emotion and spiritual being. In all honesty, I can not offer a rational conceptual framework for the formation of energy cysts in these contexts. Nonetheless, my clinical observations lead me to believe that such is the case. Once formed, the effect of the energy cyst is the same regardless of the cause.

Should an energy cyst be eradicated or released? I have heard many arguments about the positive aspects of maintaining the status quo, provided it is reasonably functional. I think that physiologically it is always desirable to release the energy cyst. However, mental and emotional factors must be taken into consideration. Is the patient ready to confront the emotion which may be involved in the release? Is he or she truly motivated? Do you, the therapist, have enough faith in the self-corrective process to stay with it wherever it may go? If yes, then go ahead. In my experience, the patient's body will tell you how much it can handle. Various methods for release of energy cysts, described later in this chapter, involve such techniques as gentle traction of the fasciae involved, passage of healing energy by the V-spread technique and somatoemotional release.

B. Facilitated segments

This concept is relevant to neuromusculoskeletal as well as psychoemotional problems. Usually, the word "facilitated" has a positive connotation, implying that some process is made easier or more efficient. In the case of the "facilitated segment," however, it means that the stimulus threshold (i.e., resistance to the conduction of an electrical impulse) in a particular spinal cord segment has been reduced. This means that the facilitated segment of the spinal cord is highly excitable, and that a smaller stimulus will trigger impulse firing in the segment.

This hypersensitivity may be detrimental to the body as a whole, depending on the tissues involved. For example, if the segment which innervates the stomach becomes facilitated, the stomach becomes hypersensitive. Therefore, mildly irritating food substances may cause disproportionately large pains and/or stomach dysfunctions. The person who has this problem may be said to have a nervous stomach or to possess food allergies or intolerances. If the situation continues, gastritis or ulceration may follow.

The concept of the facilitated segment originated in work done by Dr. I.M. Korr and his associates, beginning in the 1940's at the Kirksville College of Osteopathy and Surgery. The word "segment" means one of the parts into which something separates or divides. In the phrase "facilitated segment," the word can be somewhat misleading. It suggests that the spinal cord is naturally divided into pieces or segments. To some extent, this is true, but we must keep in mind that the spinal cord is a longitudinal structure, both functionally and structurally. It connects the brain with the nerve roots, which branch out to form the peripheral nervous system. The spinal cord can be analogized to a freeway, and the spinal nerve roots to on-ramps and off-ramps. Although the spinal cord is a continuous structure, the nerve roots do branch off at regular intervals, and can thus be viewed as delimiting "segments" of the spinal cord.

A spinal segment, in this sense, can be defined as a level of the spinal cord at which two dorsal nerve roots (sensory) enter and two ventral nerve roots (motor) exit. In a facilitated segment, these roots are overly sensitive, or hair-triggered, as explained above. The hyperactive ventral motor root from the segment passes through the intervertebral foramen and joins the sympathetic nerve chain, which thereby comes under constant bombardment. This in turn keeps the sympathetic nervous system in a state of chronic overactivity, resulting ultimately in damage to the target organs and the patient's health. If the "trophic nerve function" hypothesis is true (SEE GLOSSARY), this process may also result in protein deprivation in the target organs.

A facilitated segment produces a palpable change in tissue texture. The local paravertebral muscles and connective tissues develop a "shoddy" feel, and joints in the area are less mobile. The tissues are tender to the touch and often painfully irritable. I believe that the term "fibrositis" (SEE GLOSSARY) can be applied to the connective tissues in this situation. Sympathetic system dysfunction at the level of the facilitated segment also produces changes in skin texture, sweat gland activity and capillary blood supply to the skin.

Dr. Korr compares the facilitated segment to a "neuronal lens." By this he means that it seems to gather nerve impulses. It does not pass on its sensory input; rather, it accumulates and hoards not only those stimuli which come into it directly, but also those which are attempting to pass through to other segments. Experimental electromyographic work done by Dr. Korr and his associates has demonstrated that increased stimulus of the nervous system almost anywhere will result in increased electrical activity of the muscles serviced by nerve roots derived from a facilitated segment.

Facilitated segments seem to occur at areas of focus for postural stress, sites of trauma, and segmental levels related to visceral problems. Once established, a facilitated segment can continue for years, even contributing ultimately to death. A facilitated segment at T4 may cause decreased vitality of the heart, leading to blockage of coronary arteries and myocardial infarction. A facilitated segment tends to perpetuate itself. That is, the hyperactivity of the motor root causes the related sympathetic ganglion to become hyperactive, leading to dysfunction and deterioration of the target organs. A variety of sensory stimuli related to the dysfunction are sent back to the spinal segment, further increasing its level of facilitation, and so on. Different types of problems are associated with facilitated segments at specific levels, e.g., T9/10 (gall bladder), T12/L1 (kidney), L5 (urogenital), etc. (SEE "SEGMENTAL RELATIONSHIPS" in GLOSSARY.) Once a segment becomes facilitated, all of the associated target structures (connective tissue, muscle, bone, blood vessels, skin, sweat glands and internal organs) will be adversely affected.

Therapeutically, any approach which interrupts the self-perpetuating activity of the facilitated segment will be helpful. The sensory input to the segment must be reduced. Effective approaches, therefore, include those which: (1) relax the muscles (massage, soft tissue manipulation); (2) mobilize the area and thus reduce stasis and edema (structural manipulative therapy); (3) reduce postural stress (rolfing, Alexander technique); (4) reduce the number of signals from higher centers of the central nervous system (relaxation techniques, biofeedback, hypnotherapy, psychotherapy, tranquilizers); (5) combine these effects (osteopathic manipulative treatment). Craniosacral therapy is also very helpful in that it reduces autonomic tone (sympathetic activity), reduces general stress and anxiety, helps endocrine function, assists in postural balancing and improves fluid exchange.

C. Interference waves/arcing technique

According to my concept, interference waves are waves of energy constantly produced by an active pathological process in the body. The energy cyst is one possible source. I use the word "interference" to describe these waves because they seem superimposed upon the normal rhythmic, wave-like activity of the craniosacral system which is palpable on the human body. I perceive the waves as arcing movements which go back and forth at variable rates for different people. Occasionally, their frequency is the same as the normal craniosacral rhythm. Usually it is faster, but seldom is it greater than 60 cycles per minute.

Depending upon the distance of your hands from the lesion, you may palpate arcs of different acuteness with each hand. The "arc" is the motion perceived by your hand, visualized as an arc on the surface of an imaginary globe. Your task is to estimate the center point of this globe. You have as many tries as you wish, from as many different directions and distances as you desire. The closer you get, the tighter the arc becomes. Thus, you can zero in on the center of the globe (i.e., the lesion generating the interference waves).

Arcing is the technique used to locate energy cysts and other active pathological conditions. This technique seems to cause confusion among students. I use it in the same way I do the dural tube technique (SECTION II.F). Once you are able to focus your attention upon the patient's body motions and successfully discover the arcs, you should be able to "see" their source in your mind's eye. I believe the arcing technique gives you a chance to zero in with your intuitive powers, and provides a "crutch" to use if you have trouble believing that diagnostic intuition really works. Aside from this brief note, I have nothing to add to the description of this technique found in my first book (UPLEDGER 1983:244-50).

D. Significance detector

The term "significance detector" refers to use of the craniosacral system by the examiner to discover body positions and thought processes which are relevant to the subject's dysfunction or problem. When the body position is exactly correct for the release of an energy cyst, or for somatoemotional release, the craniosacral rhythm suddenly stops. This is not the gentle, gradual lull induced by most craniosacral techniques (such as the CV4), but more like a screeching halt. The rhythm also stops abruptly when the subject speaks of or thinks about an issue which is emotionally significant. Hence the term "significance detector." If the rhythm does not stop, you are not working in a significant (physical or emotional) area.

E. Localized diagnosis

Fascial mobility is easily evaluated by examining the physiological movement of the fascia under the urging of the craniosacral system. If there is a lack of motion symmetry in any location or for any reason, fascial mobility is restricted. In this situation, a manual evaluation of fascial glide will enable you to zero in on the exact location of the restriction. Frequently, this will be an energy cyst or the residue of an old injury or pathology. Active pathologies send out interference waves and can be detected by the arcing technique; old ones cannot. This fact allows the practitioner to differentiate active from inactive lesions or pathologies.

Skin texture changes produced by a facilitated segment are also palpable as you lightly drag your fingers over the nearby paravertebral area of the back. I usually do skin drag evaluation moving from the top of the neck to the sacral area in one motion. Where your fingertips drag on the skin, you will probably find the facilitated segment. After several repetitions, with increased force, the affected area will appear redder than nearby areas. This is the "red reflex." Muscles and connective tissues at this level will: (1) have a "shoddy" feel (like BB's under the skin); (2) be more tender to palpation; (3) be tight and tend to restrict vertebral motion; and (4) exhibit tenderness of the spinous processes when tapped by fingers or a rubber hammer.

An obstruction of the meridians of acupuncture by energy cysts is easily palpable. It is necessary that you familiarize yourself with the fourteen primary meridians and their direction of flow. With a little practice, you will be able to sense, by gently placing your hands on the patient's skin, where the obstruction is. Before the chi reaches the obstruction, the meridian will feel full (possibly also hot, or hard), like a garden hose turned on at the faucet but closed at the nozzle. Beyond the obstruction, the meridian will feel empty (and possibly cold).

Chinese pulse diagnosis can assist in this situation. Pulse diagnosis is a diagnostic technique whereby the twelve major organ systems are assigned individual pulse positions on the body. The most commonly used artery is the radial artery at the wrist; however, I have seen acupuncturists use the dorsal pedis pulses of the foot in much the same way. After you release the energy cyst or other obstruction and restore the flow of chi along the meridian, the Chinese pulses will immediately change toward normal. I have been privileged to work with several experienced acupuncture practitioners at our health center, and they have confirmed this observation.

I have also become reasonably adept at palpating what I interpret to be the flow of microcurrents of electricity on or in the body. Palpation at the ankles, feet, wrists and hands is especially easy. One can feel these currents begin to flow as energy cysts and fascial restrictions are released. They seem to flow from the center of the body to the periphery.

A long time ago, Dr. Zri Karni and I spent hours discussing body electricity. We finally agreed on the likelihood that fascia acts as a specialized conductor for microcurrents. Dr. Karni also agreed, back in the 1970's, that I was feeling these currents with my hands. He made an appointment at the "shielded room" at MIT with a friend of his to do some preliminary studies with "palpable" microcurrents, but his visiting professorship was not renewed and he had to return to Israel before we could perform the experiments. Becker (1985) describes in a detailed, scientific manner what appears to be the same phenomenon I have observed.

F. Whole body diagnosis

The techniques described in the preceding section can also be applied in whole body diagnosis. In addition, you can use the craniosacral rhythm (rate per minute) to identify tissues (usually muscles) in which the trophic nerve function has been compromised. The deprived tissue will exhibit a rate of about 25 cycles per minute. After treatment, the rate should synchronize with the normal craniosacral rhythm as palpated on the head.

The dural tube is the extension of the craniosacral system between the foramen magnum and the sacrococcygeal complex, where it is anchored to the coccyx as its periosteum. If you traction the dural tube very gently, so as not to recruit extradural muscle resistance, you can project your mind down the tube to discover resistance to easy motion. After a few hours' experience, you will find that traction is not even necessary; you can simply project your mind down the tube and "know" things about the patient. What you "know" seems related to which questions you have in mind during the examination. You can tell which segments are facilitated and even "see" the cause of the facilitation. You can also "see" membrane restriction, conditions within the dural tube, and even into the sleeves which project out to cover the spinal nerve roots. Using the dural tube as your starting point, you learn to visualize the primary causes of patients' problems quite accurately. The other techniques described can confirm your impressions.

Once you have located a facilitated segment with the dural tube technique, sit the patient up and examine for tissue change, mobility loss and "red reflex." Place a finger on each side of the spinous process at the affected level. Place the flattened palm and fingers of the other hand lightly over the front of the body at the same level and follow the motion that occurs. The tissues will begin to move back and forth. Gradually you will feel the restricted vertebrae mobilize. It will feel as though you are rolling a barrel hoop around the patient's body. Eventually you will feel a release similar to that which you feel when releasing one of the transverse diaphragms. At this point, reevaluate for the presence of the facilitated segment; it may be gone. If it is still present, repeat the process. Finally, reevaluate the dural tube; the facilitation should be gone from there too. If not, repeat the process. You take away the secondary effects first, and then the underlying cause. It seems that when the anterior body releases first, the problem was somatovisceral, and the opposite is true for viscerosomatic problems. This is probably because the viscera are anatomically anterior to vertebral somatic dysfunctions (SEE "REFLEX" in GLOSSARY). The general principle for all release techniques is "first in, last out."

I like to correct a facilitated segment in this gentle way because it does not intrude on the patient's body and set up resistance which might interfere with further diagnosis after the segment has been released. I use intrusive techniques only when I know more subtle diagnostic techniques won't be needed later during that session. The same technique can be used within the skull. Visualize and discover the problem. Place a hand on the restricted bone, the other hand opposite, and encourage movement to the release point. It is truly a beautiful experience to treat a head this way.

I seldom use techniques other than the dural tube and arcing anymore; it doesn't seem necessary. But then, I have admitted to myself that these are intuitive phenomena which I can not explain scientifically. I am not afraid of them, and I trust myself, which is probably the most important part of the whole process.

G. Regional unwinding or somatoemotional release

This technique deals with a known injury. It doesn't matter when the injury occurred; the patient is still suffering its effects. Let's suppose the patient suffered an injury to the right shoulder in a skiing accident five year ago. Since then the patient has periodically experienced shoulder pain with restricted movement. In the course of an examination using the techniques described in section II.F., you discover an upper thoracic facilitated segment. You begin treatment by placing the patient in either the sitting or standing position. You then fully support the shoulder and arm with your hands so that the muscles of the shoulder girdle are free to move as though the total arm and shoulder were weightless. You follow the motion that results from this simulated weightlessness. Sometimes a very slight traction or compression is needed to get things moving; which one depends on the vector of the original injury. You must be very sensitive to the arm's slightest inclination, following it to a position where the muscle and fascial tensions minus gravity (which you are nullifying) are perfectly balanced. This point of balanced tension (or position of balance) is dynamic; you must be alert and keep moving with it. When the precisely correct position is reached, the craniosacral rhythm stops abruptly. This is one way in which the rhythm is used as a significance detector.

At this point your hands supporting the shoulder and arm become immovable until the rhythm begins again with a concerted motion, and the shoulder and arm have at least partially softened or released. If an energy cyst releases, you will feel a dissipation of heat. It is important not to let the arm move, even though it seems so inclined, until the process (softening, release of heat, etc.) is complete and the craniosacral rhythm has resumed with a healthy amplitude. Sometimes, the arm may move only a fraction of an inch after release, and then the craniosacral rhythm stops again. In this case, prevent further movement until another release is complete and the rhythm resumes. This start/stop process may repeat itself several times before the injury is completely discharged from the area. When the full treatment is over, the patient's whole body will relax and he or she will know that it is over.

If there is emotional energy locked in the energy cyst, it will come out during the treatment process. I used the skiing injury example because I recently had such a patient. It took about three treatments, but the emotional part finally emerged. She was still very angry at the skier who had cut in front of her on the downhill slope, causing her to fall, and who didn't even stop to see if she was hurt. This anger was locked deeply inside, probably in the energy cyst that was released.

After the release, she breathed rapidly and began to talk about the incident. As she did, her craniosacral rhythm stopped until she got in touch with the extent of her anger, which was still present five years after the event. Once that anger was discharged (and she consciously forgave the offending skier), all was well with her physical body and the vestiges of the accident were fully dissipated.

To use somatoemotional release, it is important that you be confident in your ability to sense the craniosacral rhythm. Beginners in this technique should work with release of diaphragms and facilitated segments, and later with regional unwinding. After this skill is developed, the therapist is ready for whole body somatoemotional release technique.

H. Whole body somatoemotional release

During the past five years, I have added significantly to my experience in somato-emotional release techniques. There is no realistic way to separate somatoemotional release into diagnostic and therapeutic components. Similarly, you cannot separate body-work from mind-work. The mind and body are one, like the head and tail of a coin. The head is obvious on one side and the tail on the other. How deep do you penetrate into the head before it becomes the tail?

The difference between regional and whole body somatoemotional release is that in the former you let the patient consciously decide what you are going after. In the latter case, neither of you consciously knows where you are headed. It is like a "whole person scan" to discover residual somatoemotional hangups.

I can't tell you how somatoemotional release works. I know that the intention of the therapist has a lot to do with it. Also, the less guarded the patient is, the quicker it will work; I have seen the process break down in determined people who had decided to resist. Although it can be performed one-on-one, the technique is easier and more relaxed when more than one therapist is working.

When working one-on-one, I still use the standing, sitting and lying down positions described in my first book, but now I can usually "see" in advance the position which will give the release. I therefore can position myself and the patient properly to facilitate the process, saving time and trouble.

In multiple-therapist somatoemotional release, one person must be in charge; the others act as his or her extensions. If an assistant begins acting independently, a therapeutic method conflict is likely to follow, with the patient as the battleground. Decide on who will be in charge before therapy begins. The leader should tune in to the patient's body, starting at the head. As he or she senses areas of restriction, the assistants are stationed accordingly. The leader then senses the presence of the assistants at each station, as well as the effects of their therapy. He or she then regulates the amount of energy that each assistant is putting in or taking out, in order to achieve the desired release. There can be as many assistants as the leader can effectively manage.

You begin putting energy into the patient with the intention that he (or she) will release whatever he shouldn't have inside. Keep your hands on the body, follow where they lead and be alert to stops in craniosacral rhythm. When a stop occurs, hold that position no matter how hard the body tries to escape. Don't let the body move until the craniosacral rhythm resumes with renewed vitality. Then follow the movement of the patient's body until the rhythm stops again, and so on, until a full release is perceived. Encourage the patient to release emotionally. Use the craniosacral rhythm as a significance detector. You can interrupt the session at any time that the rhythm is occurring normally, and pick up very nearly where you left off in another session, up to two weeks later.

It seems impossible to overtreat using these methods, because if the subject is balanced and free of restrictions, there is nothing to treat. Sessions should not be scheduled more than two weeks apart, as this may lead to some regression, or at least a loss of momentum. Do not interrupt a session while the rhythm is stopped, as this will leave the patient "hung up" and intensify his or her physical and emotional distress.

Since we began using this therapeutic process, we have observed that the subject's body seems to be of two "minds." One part wants to maintain the status quo. After all, the body is working, even if some pain or restriction is present. Why risk a change? And yet another part is striving for improvement or loss of discomfort, which means that the energy cyst must be dissipated. During the process of somatoemotional release, we act as facilitators in cooperation with that part of the subject that wants to dissipate the energy cyst. In order to do this, we encourage the positive aspects of the body/mind and discourage the negative aspects. This involves facilitating the body's memory of the injury and thus ending the suppression.

This facilitation is accomplished by touching the subject, tuning in to what the positive body would like to do and assisting in the process. The usual result is that the body assumes the position it was in when the injury occurred. As this happens, we feel the tissues relax as the energy cyst is expelled. We also feel heat radiating from the areas which have been retaining the cyst, and frequently sense a force leaving the body along the same vector by which the injury entered.

This process requires extreme sensitivity on the part of the therapist, and an attitude of trust and positivity on the part of the patient. During the session, the release of the energy cyst frequently results in a re-experiencing of the pain, fear, anguish, anger or resentment involved in the original accident. This may occur immediately, or within the next few hours or days. It is a good sign that the treatment has released a part, if not all, of the retained problem. When this occurs, the patient should not try to suppress the pain or emotion. He or she should concentrate on the memory and try to re-experience it as fully as possible; when this is accomplished, he must then eradicate the destructive negativity and convert it to positive, constructive energy. The process of somatoemotional release is not always pleasant, but the results are worth the effort.

This is a type of therapy that has to be experienced to be appreciated. It is surprisingly powerful, often cutting directly to the heart of the matter. A few pointers:

- Questioning of patients is not so much for information as to stimulate self-realization. Don't persistently question except for this purpose. Be sensitive.
- Discharge of "negative" emotion is always good. As the therapist, be careful not to become an ally to the patient's anger and righteous indignation. Don't agree that it wasn't fair, etc., because that only fuels the formation of more anger.
- Stress that the only way to get well is by forgiving the people with whom the patient is angry. Forgiveness must be emotional as well as intellectual. You will feel the body softening as this happens.
- Frequently the patient can "image" anger, hurt, etc. If so, have him localize it and push it out into your hand. Have him look for "roots" of the "ball of anger" before it is completely out. If there are roots, have him follow them to their source with his mind's eye and gently pull them out as well. The root source may suggest another aspect of the problem requiring further work.
- It may be preferable for the patient to "somatize" an illness rather than to take it away from the body. Inappropriate and forced removal of somatization may force an emotional confrontation which you are ill-equipped to handle. You may need help from another professional before the patient can confront the truth.
- Be aware of your attitude and the tone of your voice. Be supportive and caring. If you don't feel that way, gracefully end the session.
- Do not encourage intellectualization. This takes the subject out of his right brain and can override the truth that can be offered through the body.

- Don't use too much physical force. Be firm but not forceful. Excessive force interferes with the subject's own somatic and emotional processes.
- Don't get involved in the therapist-patient hierarchy. Therapeutically it is counter-productive, because in this work the therapist is only a facilitator.
- Distraction can result from excessive patting or solicitude, as well as from talking. Distraction is harmful as it interrupts the process.
- Try to end the session by getting the patients to laugh at themselves.

III. LOCALIZED TISSUE INTELLECT, MEMORY AND EMOTION

Since I've been doing this work, I've become increasingly aware that body regions, energy cysts, tissues and perhaps individual cells all have their own intelligence, memory and emotion. These localized "brains" may not always be in communication with our conscious awareness, or even with the subconscious centers of the central nervous system.

This concept of auxiliary brains occurred to me fairly recently. First, I thought of the trigeminal ganglion as an auxiliary brain, i.e., a lot of information comes into that ganglion. It may be processed there, or triage decisions may be made in the ganglion and action taken upon the decision without requiring central nervous system input. Then I listened to my friend Michael Patterson, Ph.D. (Director of Research at Ohio University, College of Osteopathic Medicine) expound on his research which showed that decerebrate laboratory rats could solve food-oriented maze problems. This work suggested that the spinal cord has memory, can make decisions and solve problems. This was an entirely new concept for me. An issue of the *Brain Mind Bulletin* (1985) described work that showed decision-making occurring in the hands of musicians without central nervous system input. This coincided with my own experience as a jazz musician. I think craniosacral therapists' hands can work autonomously as well. Hence, my concept of auxiliary brains in the hands, spinal cord and in many of the ganglia throughout the body. Perhaps these powers develop in these peripheral locations in response to a person's need to develop certain skills.

How many of you body workers do your best work when you just give your hands free reign to do what they want? Perhaps you are distracted and see later that you have done something with the patient without having consciously decided to do it. I have this experience almost daily. I used to think I was letting my lower brain, or my right brain, do the job. But perhaps my hands simply do the job without guidance from the spinal cord, or any other part of the central nervous system.

In my reckless youth, I made a living as a jazz piano player. I became able to study books and notes (I was a university student) while I was playing piano at a dance or in a cocktail lounge. The other musicians said they couldn't tell the difference in my playing, except that I was a little "looser" when I was studying something else and playing piano at the same time. I frequently had to be reminded by a drumstick tap on the shoulder when the end of the song was coming; otherwise I might continue into another chorus after the other musicians had stopped. Eventually my hands seemed to become totally independent. I had to watch them to see what they were playing. For example, if the bass player asked me which chord I had played during a certain measure, I had to replay that part of the song and watch my fingers in order to answer him. It seemed that my hands had their own intelligence and were independent of the higher brain centers.

An interesting book on this topic was given to me recently (SUDNOW 1978). The author, David Sudnow, was a sociology professor at City University of New York, and a jazz piano player. The book describes the process of learning the art of jazz improvisation, and the development of the autonomy of his hands. As he became more accomplished, he felt like a third-party observer as his hands played the music.

What does all this have to do with somatoemotional release and the other techniques described in section II? Perhaps we have independent intelligences in each part of our body, with memory of trauma, emotion, etc. Perhaps by means of these techniques we are helping these "micro-intelligences" to escape from the emotional and somatic scars they are carrying. The ramifications of this idea are truly mind-boggling. At any rate, the techniques work very well, and I will continue to use them. I hope that you will too.

AFTERWORD

Many students have inquired about my own belief system and how things fit together for me. They have asked me "where I am" spiritually. I have decided to write this Afterword in an attempt to answer these questions.

I think each of us has a spirit, soul, or higher self (as you prefer) which tells our subconscious mind what needs to be done with our life. Within our mind is a censor or filter system which prevents us from being consciously aware of this message and our purpose. After all, if you read the end of a mystery story first, what's the point? If we are to learn a lesson from our lifetime, it might be counter-productive to know why everything happened as it did, in advance.

Our mind lives in our brain and expresses its requests to the brain, which then passes the orders along to the rest of the central nervous system. The central nervous system in turn delegates duties to its somatic and autonomic divisions. The somatic division tells the musculoskeletal system what needs to be done. The autonomic division tells the viscera what they must do in order to enable the muscles, bones and joints to do their jobs. In the final analysis it is the musculoskeletal system that executes the commands of the mind. The mind is pretty much unaware of the impositions made upon the various support systems in the process of carrying out its orders.

All in all it looks like my higher self wants me to do something with this lifetime on earth. It has taken title to this body as a vehicle and a means of getting the job done.

GLOSSARY OF
TERMS AND CONCEPTS

Autogenic pain: Pain which is self-perpetuating. The mechanism of this type of pain is usually neural-mechanical. For an example involving the jugular foramen and sternocleidomastoid, see chapter 1, section IX and chapter 3, section VIII.

Autonomic ganglia: Aggregations of nerve cell bodies related to the autonomic nervous system and located outside of the central nervous system. These ganglia direct nerve impulses in proper directions after information comes in from the sensory end organs. They appear to make some decisions without relying on higher centers of the central nervous system. For this reason I think of them as "auxiliary brains" (CHAPTER 4, SECTION III).

The *celiac ganglion* is located on the aorta and provides sympathetic innervation to the stomach, liver, pancreas, spleen and adrenal medulla.

The *mesenteric ganglia,* superior and inferior, are located adjacent to the abdominal aorta (at the bifurcation) in the mid and lower abdominal cavity. They have sympathetic function, receiving preganglionic fibers from spinal nerve roots T10 through L1. Their postganglionic sympathetic motor fibers are distributed to the small intestine, large intestine, kidneys, urinary bladder and sex organs.

The *sympathetic ganglia* are located periodically along the length of the sympathetic chains bilaterally between the upper cervical and the upper lumbar regions. The sympathetic nervous system arises from intermediolateral cell columns of the spinal cord between T1 and L3-4. The ventral roots exit the spinal cord and reach the sympathetic trunk ganglia via the white communicating rami. Usually they synapse within the ganglia, but may do so after travelling up or down the sympathetic chain. After synapsing, the postganglionic fibers are distributed to all viscera and blood vessels of the body.

1. The *cervical sympathetic ganglia* are located bilaterally next to the cervical vertebrae. There are three divisions (superior, middle and inferior), connected vertically by the fibers of the cervical sympathetic chain. These chains are located within the fascia of the carotid sheaths on each side of the vertebrae just anterior to the trans-

verse processes. The superior cervical sympathetic ganglion is described in chapter 1, section III.L. The middle cervical sympathetic ganglion, the smallest of the three divisions, is usually located at the level of the C6-7, and is sometimes called the thyroid ganglion or vertebral ganglion. It communicates with spinal nerves C5, C6 and sometimes C4. Its branches often follow the vertebral arteries, join the cardiac plexi, service the thyroid gland and follow the subclavian arteries. The inferior cervical sympathetic ganglion is located between the base of the transverse process of C7 and the neck of the first rib. It is often fused with the first thoracic sympathetic ganglion, in which case it is called the stellate ganglion. It communicates with spinal nerve C6 and follows the vertebral artery as the artery enters the foramen to ascend into the head. There is also communication with C7, C8 and the inferior cardiac plexus.

2. The *thoracic sympathetic ganglia* are the thoracic counterparts of the cervical sympathetic ganglia described above. The upper thoracic sympathetic ganglion, as noted, may be fused to the inferior cervical sympathetic ganglion, in which case it is called the stellate ganglion.

Other autonomic ganglia, described in chapter 1, include: ciliary (SECTION III.E.1), geniculate (SECTION V.D), inferior vagal (SECTION VIII.B), jugular (SECTION VIII.B), otic (SECTION V.H), sphenopalatine (SECTIONS III.M and V.G), submaxillary (SECTION IV.D), and vestibular (SECTION VI.B.1).

Autonomic nervous system: The autonomic nervous system is the normally involuntary or "unconscious" division of the peripheral nervous system. It is efferent or motor to all of the smooth muscles (including those in the blood vessel walls) and to the glands and viscera. It is the autonomic nervous system's function that biofeedback seeks to bring under voluntary control, since the autonomic system has a great influence upon blood pressure, heart rate, breathing and digestive function.

The autonomic nervous system has two divisions, sympathetic and parasympathetic. They are discussed separately below.

Biofeedback: The system whereby information about physiological functions, of which the individual is largely unaware and over which he therefore exercises little voluntary control, is channeled back to the individual. Conscious awareness sometimes allows voluntary control over these functions. Alyce and Elmer Green of the Menninger Foundation are pioneers in this field. Their book, *Beyond Biofeedback,* is an excellent source for further information.

Biofeedback techniques have been used to bring voluntary control to many functions, including blood pressure, heart rate and rhythm, muscle tension and brain wave activity. The limitations of this technique seem imposed only by the mind of the therapist.

Brain development: Brain development has been thought to end early in life, and damage to the brain thought to be irreversible. My own work with brain dysfunctioning children caused me to doubt the validity of this assumption as early as 1977. In doing craniosacral therapy on so-called "dead end" or "hopeless" cases, I saw "irreversible damage" reverse itself several times. The work of Doman and Delacato, in which they describe "cross-patterning," also argues against the "irreversibility" of brain damage in some cases.

Evidence now supports the idea that brain growth continues throughout life. If one exercises the brain in much the same way that one exercises a muscle, with regular and increasing demand, that brain will respond by growing and developing further functional ability. This concept suggests that the therapist should always try to restore function, even if it seems hopeless. You never know what may happen. Many of my own successes occurred because I was too dumb to know that the case was "hopeless."

Chakras: These have been conceptualized by yogis in India since ancient times as centers of the ethereal body (energy body which engulfs the physical body) which take in vitality (prahna) from the surrounding atmosphere in order to energize the individual. In general, chakras are best palpated just off the physical body of the patient, although touching is permissible. They can range from 3-15cm in diameter. In my perception, the first six of the chakras described below are associated with energy fields which spin clockwise. There are seven chakras which are palpable to me:

The *root chakram* is related to sexuality and reproduction, and is said to be the seat of the "kundalini" (fiery serpent). Kundalini is thought to be an energy derived from the sun, stored at the base of the spine and, when liberated, to rush up the spinal canal to the brain, activating all the chakras as it passes them. I have treated a few advanced yogis who said that craniosacral therapy enhanced and made easier the ascent of their kundalini. The root chakram is palpable in the supine patient with one hand placed under the sacrum and the other, very lightly, on the lower abdomen just above the symphysis pubis. I have found this chakram to be inactive most frequently in women who have an unsatisfactory sexual life, especially those who trade sex for material support with no feeling of love. Opening this chakram and the heart chakram simultaneously will frequently improve and integrate the sexual and love relationships.

The *navel chakram* is related to sensitivity, feelings and emotions, as well as the function of the liver, kidneys, intestines, digestion and solar plexus. It is best palpated with one hand under the upper and middle lumbar spine and the other just below the navel, barely touching the body.

The *spleen chakram* is related to the assimilation of energy and its distribution to other parts of the body; it is similar to the concept found in acupuncture theory of the spleen as the refiner and distributor of chi to the other organs. This chakram is best palpated with one hand holding the thoracolumbar junction and the other placed very lightly over the epigastrium. Improving the function of this chakram will often improve immunity, resistance and general activity levels.

The *heart chakram* is best palpated with one hand under the mid-thoracic spine and the other hand just touching the mid-sternal area. In my experience, this chakram is frequently dysfunctional in persons who have been hurt, as children, by someone in whom they had great trust. Now, they are afraid to love for fear of being hurt again. As mentioned above, the heart and root chakras together are frequently dysfunctional in women whose marriages involve sex without love.

The *throat chakram* is best palpated with one hand cradling the back of the neck and the other covering the thyroid cartilage, with a thumb and finger on the two upper lateral extremities of the cartilage. Frequently, the chakram is felt as two separate energy centers, each spinning clockwise on the two sides of the throat; I believe this is normal. This chakram has to do with communication with other people, and the ability to verbally express one's feelings.

The *brow chakram* is related to: (a) the pituitary and pineal glands; (b) clairvoyance and the ability to perceive things in connection with interpersonal relationships; (c) sensing the character of other persons and the purity of their motives. The spinning of its energy field is more intense than the other chakras mentioned above. I usually palpate it with one hand (optional) under the occiput and two or three finger tips over the glabella.

The *crown chakram* is palpable with one hand at the vertex of the head. I seldom perceive it as spinning, but rather as on outflow of energy which increases as the patient's energy is enhanced. It is also said to be related to the pineal gland, or to have a spiritual or cosmic connection.

I treat chakras by thinking hard and visualizing what they are supposed to be doing; believe it or not, they usually do it. Often, emotional release accompanies improvement in chakra function.

Conflict: Synonyms for this word include collision, disagreement, clash, opposition, contention, controversy, etc. It is significant that there are so many synonyms. We see conflict in societies as well as individuals.

In health care, we observe many people who seek conflict, both internally and externally. They are the tough competitors, the angry, the vindictive, and so on. The conflict is destructive to their health and well-being, but on the other hand it seems to be the fuel that keeps them going. Similarly, human society seems historically to have thrived on war.

Consciousness: I use this term to mean awareness, on an individual, group or universal level. "Universal consciousness" denotes the cosmic pool of knowledge which believers say is available to those who will take the time to tap into it. The "eurekas!" or insights which we have are thought by some to be temporary connections with the universal mind or consciousness.

Craniosacral system: Because this entire book (and my earlier one) are about craniosacral therapy, it might seem a bit strange to include a glossary entry about the subject. However, I think it is important to at once put everything in perspective, in a nutshell. I conceptualize the craniosacral system as the place where mind, body and spirit come together. What does this mean? That by going through the craniosacral system, by using it as a handle, you can learn about and influence these three aspects of human life.

An example of this is the "significance detector" (CHAPTER 4, SECTION II.D). A sudden stop in the craniosacral rhythm can indicate a significant position of the body (the correct position for the release of an energy cyst), or an event that is significant for the mind or spirit, although consciously unimportant to the patient.

There are also ways in which the craniosacral system may have a direct influence on important, on-going physiological processes. For example, the continuing rhythmical movement of the craniosacral system may serve to "milk" the pituitary gland, with all the implications this would hold for the neuroendocrine system. It is possible that this rhythmical motion is also an important stimulus for proper development of the brain. Similarly, the motion around the skull sutures may pump the newly-formed red blood cells out of the flat bones of the skull and into the general circulation.

One thing that the many hours I have spent in intimate contact with the craniosacral system has taught me is that it is indeed very close to the center of life. As an illustration of what I mean, let me relate what happened to my friend June MacRae, an osteopathic physician, when she entered the hospital room of one of her patients who had a terminal metastatic malignancy. At the time the patient was in terminal respiratory distress. Dr. MacRae began some gentle craniosacral balancing. The patient relaxed. The craniosacral system went into a great flexion, hesitated for a moment, and then went into extension. The patient died quietly at that moment.

Crisis intervention: This term describes the type of health care applied after the patient's health has deteriorated to a level at which symptoms interfere with body functions and may be life-threatening. Crisis intervention is the antithesis of preventive health care. It ends when the crisis is no longer apparent, and does not seek the cause or attempt to prevent later crises.

Endogenous therapeutic biochemicals: The founder of osteopathic medicine, over 100 years ago, was Andrew Taylor Still. One of his primary tenets was, "The body makes its own medicine." He was just a bit ahead of his time. We know now that the human body has a whole pharmacopoeia of molecules which it can manufacture as indicated for various conditions. The beauty of these endogenous therapeutic biochemicals is that they are essentially free to the user, no prescription is required and they are usually without untoward side effect.

Among these therapeutic agents are the antibodies which we produce to neutralize and/or destroy specific pathogens, the endorphins and encephalins which modify pain sensations and the almost endless list of other neuropeptides which influence everything from the immune system to appetite.

Fibrositis: The concept of fibrositis has been with us since 1904, when the term was introduced by Sir William Gowers, a British physician. It is also known as myofibrositis, nonarticular rheumatism and muscular rheumatism. Around 1920, a physician named Stockman theorized that fibrositis must have an inflammatory component. However, microscopic studies of biopsies of "fibrositis tissues" have not confirmed the presence of an inflammatory component.

The symptoms of this condition are muscle spasm, pain and stiffness with restricted motion. The symptoms worsen after either prolonged disuse or overuse. The most common areas affected are the cervical, upper thoracic and lumbosacral areas of the back, as well as the shoulders and gluteal area. There seems to be a relationship between psychoemotional stress and the exacerbation of fibrositis. There are usually trigger points associated with fibrositis. These are the basis for some of the Travell's triggers, Chapman's reflexes, the tsubo of shiatsu, acupuncture points and many other such therapeutic constructs and modalities.

I believe that fibrositis and the facilitated segment concept are linked; if either persists for long it will cause the other to occur. Thus, the treatments described in chapter 4 for the facilitated segment will be effective in the treatment of fibrositis as well.

Field orientation: Becker (1985) discusses this concept. He believes that many organisms have crystalline structures within their bodies which act as magnetic field detectors, providing a sense of orientation in relationship to the earth. Such structures have been found in the ethmoid bone of pigeons. This type of orientation system is better developed in birds (which often have to fly long distances) than in humans. Humans rely on other clues for orientation; perhaps the system has undergone disuse atrophy.

Focal suicide: This concept, developed by Karl Menninger, refers to a suicidal impulse focused on a specific part of the body. Examples are forms of self-mutilation such as nail-biting, finger chewing, skin picking, etc. This idea is consistent with the concept of limited autonomy of body parts, discussed in chapter 4, section III.

Healing hands: The concept underlying this phrase is that there is a healing energy (which I believe to be electromagnetic in nature) which can be directed through the hands of one individual into the body of another for the purpose of facilitating physical (and perhaps mental or emotional) healing. The V-spread technique, and many others, are examples of this phenomenon. Work done by me and others (e.g., BECKER 1985) lends some scientific credibility to the idea. I have seen so many clinical instances of this phenomenon that I have come to accept it as matter-of-fact.

Health: This word has two definitions of interest: (1) the general condition of the body or mind, with reference to soundness and vigor; (2) freedom from disease or ailment. It is interesting that modern medicine has most often elected to use the latter definition over the past century, particularly after the development of "germ theory." It is only recently that some mainstream health professionals have looked at health as a positive commodity.

When I use the term health, I mean physiological resourcefulness and adaptability as well as soundness and vigor. I think of health as the amount of available energy needed for constructive endeavor, as well as for adaption and self-protection. I also consider how readily the individual is able to replace such energy.

Instinct: Innate (i.e., non-learned) behavior. Instinctive behavior related to courtship, mating, migration, hunting and so on are easily observed in a variety of animals. Instinctive behavior, though often camouflaged by learned "civilized behavior," is still present in humans and often guides our actions. Examples are territorial, aggressive, phobic and altruistic behavior.

Meridians of acupuncture: These are channels which have been plotted in and on the body which permit the flow of vital life energy (chi). Through them, various organs can be energized or can release abnormally high amounts of energy.

There are twelve major meridians related to internal organs. Of these, six are yin and six are yang. Two of the yin meridians (heart and pericardium) and two of the yang meridians (small intestine and triple warmer) are associated with the element fire. The other eight meridians and their associations are as follows: spleen (earth/yin), stomach (earth/yang), lung (air/yin), large intestine (air/yang), kidney (water/yin), urinary bladder (water/yang), liver (wood/yin), gall bladder (wood/yang). In addition, there are two major meridians which represent yin and yang: the conception and governing vessels, respectively.

Myofascial release: A method of manipulative treatment aimed at the relaxation of the soft tissues of the body. It focuses on muscles and fasciae that are abnormally tense or contracted, and involves the use of pressure and stretching on those tissues to relax/release them.

Pain: This is a difficult term to define. Most dictionaries describe pain as a bodily suffering or distress due to injury or illness, or as a mental or emotional torment of some kind. The problem is that pain is a subjective experience which is highly individualized, carrying with it a wide range of emotional overlay. It can be described by the sufferer only by comparing it to some other sensation which he has experienced. Thomas Lewis, writing in the early 1940's, divided pain into the sharp pain of ectodermal origin and the less localized internal ache or pain which comes from the deeper tissues of mesodermal origin. This interesting concept suggests that there are two systems of pain perception.

Controversy still exists about whether all pain impulses come into the spinal cord via the dorsal roots, or whether some input is via the anterior roots. In either case, pain impulses cross to the opposite side of the spinal cord soon after making entry. Once the crossover is complete, the impulses ascend to the thalamus via the spinothalamic tracks. Most pain pathways terminate in the thalamus, though some continue to the cortex for conscious awareness.

Health care professionals have developed numerous techniques for the blocking of pain awareness: anesthetic and analgesic agents, surgical procedures, physical therapy, consciousness altering techniques, peripheral stimulation therapy, psychotherapy, etc.

Considering the time, effort and money that have gone into pain reduction, it is obvious that we regard pain as an enemy. Although I do not endorse the cultivation of an enjoyment of pain, we should recognize that pain is an ally in that it tells you when something in your body or mind is wrong and requires attention. The key to benefitting from pain is not to ignore it, but to discover what it is trying to tell you and do something about the cause. We should *not* try to block pain from our consciousness until we know why it is there. (SEE ALSO "REFERRED PAIN" and "SUBTHRESHOLD PAIN.")

Parasympathetic nervous system: This division of the autonomic nervous system (sometimes called the craniosacral division) arises from preganglionic cell bodies in the gray matter of the brain stem and from spinal segments S2-4. Parasympathetic distribution is limited to visceral structures, whereas sympathetic distribution is to every part of the body. With few exceptions, parasympathetic preganglionic fibers travel without synapse to the wall or near vicinity of the target organ; the postganglionic fibers are quite short. Preganglionic fibers from the cranial end of the system to the viscera below the foramen magnum are carried by the vagus system (CHAPTER 1, SECTION VIII); those within the cranial vault which innervate viscera of the head are carried by the oculomotor, facial and glossopharyngeal systems (CHAPTER 1, SECTIONS III, V and VII). The sacral division of the parasympathetic system is distributed via the pelvic nerve and hypogastric plexus to the lower intestine, pelvic viscera and genitalia.

Functionally, the parasympathetic system provides motor innervation to certain visceral structures. It is a trophotropic system, i.e., it regulates those functions which are necessary for long-term survival. It is not involved in the stress or emergency responses governed by the sympathetic system. The parasympathetic system controls the processing and absorption of food, including secretion of saliva and digestive juices. It slows the heart rate and respiratory rate, causes the pancreas, liver and gall bladder to secrete, causes the kidneys to produce urine, and so on. All the things we must do to survive are conservatively regulated by this system.

Peripheral stimulation therapy (PST): This is a phrase we coined many years ago to cover a wide range of therapeutic stimuli which are applied to the skin and/or subcutaneous tissues. The phrase was designed to be an all-encompassing category of therapy for convenience in research activities. It includes acupuncture, shiatsu, acupressure, all types of electro-stimulation (e.g., TENS and electro-acupuncture), Chapman's reflexes, reflexology, Travell's trigger therapy and any other such therapy we wanted to look at. The title has served to legitimize some methods that were considered to be weird or on the "fringe" under their own names. For example, research into acupuncture was weird in 1975, but research into PST was acceptable.

Proprioception: This is the sense of where your body is in space. In craniosacral therapy, this sense is very important in the technique of "melding" your hands into the patient's body. After your hands have become one with the patient's body and your arms are moving with them, your arms can provide you the information about what your hands are doing. This approach to craniosacral work obviates the need for your tactile sense to tell you about the patient's physiological activity. With practice, the proprioceptive sensory system becomes more accurate and reliable. It is interesting that tactile senses rely on skin (ectoderm) while proprioception relies on connective tissue (mesoderm). This may explain why this sense is so useful in craniosacral diagnosis, which concentrates on connective tissue.

Referred pain: Pain which is perceived at some distance from the location of the cause. For example, pain originating in the midcervical spinal nerve roots may be experienced in the diaphragm. Pain experienced in the testicle may actually be due to a problem, often a stone, in the kidney, pelvis and/or the ureter on the same side. Anginal pain arising from the heart muscle and/or coronary artery spasm is often experienced as pain up the neck into the jaw and/or into the left arm as far distally as the hand. Disease or dysfunction of the gall bladder is experienced as pain in that area but also radiates into the right lower thoracic paravertebral area and up into the medial border of the right scapula. Appendicitis will almost always make the tip of the twelfth rib on the right very tender to palpation. The distribution of the major divisions of the trigeminal nerve (mandibular and maxillary) can be mapped out on the face when the nerve to a tooth becomes irritated and hyperactive. The teeth may ache when the actual problem is in the sinus or some other area innervated by the same nerve trunk. As shown by these examples, specific anatomic areas of referred pain experience are considered highly suggestive of specific visceral problems. The mechanism in these cases can be explained by nervous system pathways.

The facilitated segment concept (CHAPTER 4, SECTION II.B) provides a possible explanation for referred pain. "Neural cross-talk" (Dr. I.M. Korr's term) refers to the idea that one overactive nerve trunk can spill its activity over into a neighboring nerve trunk, causing pain to be felt somewhere in the distribution of the recipient nerve trunk. A facilitated segment may also spill its excess energy over to adjacent spinal cord segments.

Drs. Korr and Retzlaff have convinced me that referred pain can be mediated by the sympathetic nervous system. This allows for the referral of experienced pain along the sympathetic arterial plexuses, and for the transfer of pain impulses from the voluntary nervous system at the junctions between the sympathetic chain ganglia and the spinal cord nerve roots. Under this hypothesis, the sympathetic system may be more than an autonomic outflow (efferent) system; it may also be involved in pain perception and in this way conduct sensory input. The eradication of severe pain by sympathectomy supports this idea.

I believe that the meridian system of acupuncture and the membrane system of craniosacral therapy can also help explain some instances of referred pain. In the evaluation of a patient using the acupuncture approach, you will often find a blockage of energy flow along a meridian which relates to a visceral pain. When you open the blocked meridian, the visceral problem is resolved. A couple of recent examples come to mind. In a patient under treatment for angina pectoris, I found an obstruction to energy flow along the heart meridian at the wrist; the obstruction seemed to have its origin in an old injury to the wrist. Opening of the acupuncture meridian has obviated the need for further medical treatment of the "heart problem." Thus, in some cases it may be a question of "referred visceral disease" rather than "referred pain." In another patient, I found that a fall on the right lower leg had resulted in an obstruction of energy flow along the stomach meridian, resulting in digestive symptoms related to pylorospasm (i.e., hyperacidity, extended retention of food in the stomach and chronic epigastric pain). This could also have resulted in real visceral disease, in this case peptic ulcer or gastritis. The stomach symptoms were alleviated by the opening of the acupuncture meridian.

The referral of pain via the craniosacral system is illustrated by an example which I have seen many times: the fall on the tailbone which results in an anteriorly flexed coccyx. This produces an abnormal tension on the dural tube (apparently) which is transmitted to the head and experienced as an occipitofrontal headache.

Can pain or dysfunction transmitted to distant parts via the acupuncture meridian system or craniosacral system properly be called "referred pain"? The term, as generally used, assumes mediation by the nervous system. As long as you appreciate the alternative possibilities, I suppose the terminology will not interfere with the use of appropriate diagnostic and treatment methods. Perhaps we should talk about neuronally referred pain, meridian referred pain and craniosacrally referred pain.

Reflex: An automatic response, usually mediated via the nervous system, which may come into conscious awareness but which frequently occurs subconsciously. A variety of nerve pathways may be involved. Types of reflexes relevant to craniosacral therapy include:

Viscerosomatic. A visceral structure affects the musculoskeletal system. An example is the gall bladder causing pain and dysfunction in the lower right thoracic paravertebral region (SEE "REFERRED PAIN"). A chronic gall bladder problem may cause musculoskeletal dysfunction as the subjectively dominant symptom.

Viscerovisceral. One viscera which is in trouble causes another viscera to become dysfunctional. A serious example is the case of herpes opthalmicus, where the problem in the afflicted eye often causes loss of vision in the other eye. Another example is pneumonitis resulting from acute gall bladder disease. In view of the facilitated segment concept, we need only look at viscera which share common or adjacent innervation to appreciate how disease in one viscera can adversely influence the other.

Viscerosympathetic. Increased sensory input from a viscera spills over into the sympathetic nervous system via the facilitated segment, resulting in hyperactivity of the sympathetic system (SEE "REFERRED PAIN"), and possibly generalized stress syndrome.

Somatovisceral. The opposite of viscerosomatic: a somatic or musculoskeletal problem feeds impulses into its spinal cord segment and causes facilitation of that segment. Visceral organs which receive outflow from that segment can then become hypersensitive and eventually dysfunctional or diseased. E.g., a trauma or chronic postural stress in the musculoskeletal system manifests as a gall bladder problem via a facilitated segment.

Somatosomatic. One structure of the musculoskeletal system causes a neuronally mediated problem in another. Again, a facilitated segment may be involved. E.g., the right trapezius muscle is strained while exercising. This muscle is innervated by the spinal accessory nerve, which is derived from spinal cord segments C3 and C4. The trapezius strain results in an overload of sensory input into the midcervical region of the spinal cord, causing some facilitation of the spinal cord segments. Motor outflow is increased and the paravertebral muscles in the midcervical region become hypertonic, which in turn causes a loss of mobility, plus pain and tenderness, of the neck. The final result may be somatic dysfunction of the midcervical region. This can happen in minutes or in days, depending on the severity of the original strain.

Somatosympathetic. Similar to viscerosympathetic, except that the origin of excessive sensory input to the sympathetic system is from a somatic structure (e.g., the trapezius strain in the example above) rather than a visceral one. The result is the same.

The common factor in these examples is the facilitated segment. All the structures innervated by the involved segment are influenced adversely by its hyperactivity. The sympathetic nervous system is stimulated into a higher level of activity, which costs the subject considerable adaptive and compensatory energy (SEE "SYMPATHETIC NERVOUS SYSTEM").

Repression: A factor interfering with psychological and somatic adaptation and adjustment. Emotional repression prevents the problem from coming into awareness, and prevents the repressed area from maturing. The "energy cyst" concept (CHAPTER 4, SECTION II.A) is an example of physical repression; the energy cyst may likewise prevent the involved area of the body from developing. Release of repressed material, whether predominantly emotional or physical, is the therapeutic objective. The emotional or physical energy used in repression would be used more constructively for other purposes.

Therapies which do not release repressed emotions or energy cysts (and resolve them) produce changes which are of questionable benefit. There is strong potential for new disorder if any additional stress to the system disturbs the newly established but still-fragile equilibrium.

Segmental relationships: The segmental relationships between the spinal cord, viscera and myofascial tissues are clinically very significant. Under the "facilitated segment" concept, everything that is innervated by such a segment may be affected adversely. Myofascial tissues are contracted and painful, and the joints to which they attach are less mobile. Blood vessels related to viscera are constricted, and the viscera are more vulnerable to disease and toxic influences. Sympathetic nerve tone goes up. The trophic influence of nerve is impaired and dystrophy may result. Conduction of energy along the acupuncture meridians is impaired, and electrical conductivity of tissues is compromised.

A variety of "reflexes" are involved in a facilitated segment situation. For example, a liver inflammation sends impulses into the related spinal segment, facilitating it and causing myofascial tissue contracture and sympathetic overactivity in turn. After a while it is difficult to tell which came first, the liver inflammation or the myofascial dysfunction. The myofascial problem, if present first, may have made the liver more vulnerable to noxious influences. No tissue dysfunction in a segmental region can remain isolated, just as no spinal cord segment is isolated from the rest of the nervous system.

The general relationships of spinal segments to viscera (controversy exists in some cases) are as follows:

1. The lungs and bronchi refer into segments T1-6. Respiratory system problems are palpable as somatic dysfunction of the spinous processes of the corresponding vertebrae, or of the nearby vertebrae C7 and T7. The vagus nerve has great influence over the respiratory system, and is often affected by problems at the jugular foramen (CHAPTER 1, SECTION VIII).

2. There is evidence that heart muscle problems may manifest as left-side somatic dysfunction with loss of vertebral mobility, spinous process tenderness, paravertebral muscle tightness and skin texture changes in the region of vertebra T4, or anywhere between T1 and T6. The vagus nerve affects cardiac rhythm, so again the jugular foramen may be involved.

3. Liver and gall bladder problems may produce similar right-side changes in joint mobility, muscle tone and skin texture in the area near vertebrae T5-11. The gall bladder will often refer up to the medial border of the right scapula as tenderness to palpation.

4. The spleen can produce similar changes in the left-side area of vertebra T11.

5. The stomach refers to the lower thoracic segments, especially T6 on the left side, producing similar problems.

6. The kidneys refer into the area of T11-12 and L1-2. The eleventh ribs will also be tender to palpation.

7. The ovaries, because of their embryological descent, refer into the T12 region.

8. The appendix, when inflamed, will produce an area of exquisite tenderness to palpation on the very tip of the twelfth rib on the right side. This referral point, in my experience, has been a reliable diagnostic aid in differentiating appendicitis from ovarian problems or lymphadenopathy in the cecal region of the bowel.

9. The intestines in general refer as somatic dysfunction into the lumbar and sacral regions.

10. The pelvic organs generally refer into the upper sacral segments.

There is individual variation in these relationships, which should not surprise you. Favorable effect on visceral function is achieved by reducing the activity level of the facilitated segment. Appropriate techniques are mentioned in chapter 4, section II.B.

Somatic (neuromuscular) gravitational maladaptive syndrome: A group of symptoms resulting from a less than optimal posture, i.e., the body has to work harder than necessary to obey CNS commands regarding position maintenance in the gravitational field. This situation requires the expenditure of extra energy to stand, walk and so on. Increased overall vulnerability to internal and external stresses results. Such body therapies as rolfing, Alexander technique and Feldenkrais focus primarily upon improving gravitational adaptational efficiency.

Stillpoint: This is a therapeutic interruption of craniosacral rhythm which allows the craniosacral system to reorganize its activity for more optimal effect upon the body. The stillpoint may be imposed from outside by a therapist or it may be a spontaneous homeostatic process. It may occur very suddenly by a precise aligning of the body in a significant position, or by the experience of a significant emotion. In this way, it can function as a "significance detector" (CHAPTER 4, SECTION II.D). The stillpoint helps to balance the symmetry of the craniosacral system and corrects many restrictions in that system in a nonspecific way. It reduces sympathetic tonus, enhances fluid exchange between physiological compartments, reduces stress, lowers fever and enhances the body defense mechanisms against pathogens. It is an efficacious, wide spectrum, natural therapeutic event.

Stress: An adversity imposed on the physiology of the body/mind complex. It may be environmental (e.g., noise or cold) or arise within the individual (e.g., anxiety, phobia or nutritional disorder). The body reaction is similar in any event, involving increased sympathetic nervous system activity and all the attendant symptoms, including adrenal hyperfunction which often produces endocrine imbalance. Hans Selye described a "triad" of chronic stress symptoms: myocardial infarction, peptic ulcer and adrenal hypertrophy. These major symptoms are often preceded by others such as hypertension, angina, pylorospasm, hypoglycemia and chronic nervous tension and anxiety.

Subthreshold pain: This is a concept which I have discussed on many occasions with Dr. Ernest Retzlaff. The idea is that when a pain stimulus has existed for some time and the cause has not been corrected, the body may use one of several means at its disposal to reduce or eliminate conscious awareness of the pain. Under these circumstances, the subject continues to spend energy in order to adapt and compensate for the problem physiologically, but is unaware of it. As a result, he suffers from chronic fatigue, depression and so on. The situation may persist until the cause is brought back into conscious awareness and treated successfully (SEE "REFERRED PAIN").

Sutural dysfunction: Loss of the normal mobility at a cranial suture, resulting from injury, chronic abnormal membranous tension or microstructure. This condition must be corrected in order to normalize craniosacral system function.

Sympathetic nervous system: The sympathetic ganglia are located in the sympathetic nerve chains situated bilaterally along the vertebral column, and in the celiac, superior and inferior mesenteric ganglia. The latter three ganglia are located next to the abdominal aorta; sympathetic fibers leading to them pass through the sympathetic chain ganglia without synapsing.

The cells of origin for the preganglionic sympathetic fibers are located in the interomedial cell columns of spinal segments T12 and L1-4. The ratio of postganglionic to preganglionic sympathetic fibers is about 32:1. Thus, a single preganglionic fiber can influence a variety of postganglionic fibers.

Postganglionic sympathetic fibers are distributed as follows:

1. Those from the superior cervical sympathetic ganglia service the head via the carotid plexuses.
2. Those from all three cervical sympathetic ganglia contribute to the cardiac plexus, which acts to accelerate myocardial activity.
3. Those from the upper five thoracic sympathetic ganglia serve the thoracic aorta in a vasomotor capacity, and contribute to posterior pulmonary plexus activity in bronchodilator capacity.
4. Those with preganglionic fibers originating from the lower seven thoracic segments synapse in the celiac and superior mesenteric ganglia, and supply the abdominal organs.
5. Those with preganglionic fibers from lumbar segments synapse in the inferior mesenteric ganglion, and then supply the lower abdominal and pelvic viscera via the hypogastric plexus.

Here are a few facts about the sympathetic system that may surprise you:

1. Most tissues in the human body have sympathetic innervation.
2. Every blood vessel has sympathetic innervation which can cause contraction.
3. Blood supply to the cerebral cortex is reduced by sympathetic stimulation.
4. By influencing blood flow and metabolic rate, the sympathetic system influences pH levels and waste removal.
5. Sympathetic stimulation will (a) reduce or even stop the healing process; (b) facilitate a spinal cord segment; (c) contribute to hypertension; (d) inhibit pituitary function; (e) if chronic, inhibit bone growth (and potentially stunt the growth of a child); and (f) if chronic, contribute to the formation of atherosclerotic plaques in arteries (thus contributing to heart attack and stroke).

Sympathetic effects on target organs are often relevant to stress syndromes and diseases. The sympathetic division can be thought of as the "big spender." It does whatever is required to save your life in a time of crisis, without concern for future survival. Replenishing the resources which were spent by the sympathetic division is the responsibility of the parasympathetic division (see above). Once overactive or hypertonic, the sympathetic system often seems to create its own stress and then responds to it by further activity. If sympathetic activity does not subside after the danger is past, you begin to destroy your own body. Facilitated segments (CHAPTER 4, SECTION II.B) contribute to sympathetic hypertonus. The reduction of chronic sympathetic hypertonus is definitely worth the effort; craniosacral therapy and biofeedback are effective methods of achieving this.

Syndrome: A group of symptoms characterizing a specific dysfunction or disease. The word may also be used to denote a set of social symptoms characterizing a societal phenomenon.

Target organ: I use this term to denote that organ, in a specific subject, which tends to be affected by overall stress. For example, if your stomach is your target organ it matters little whether you wreck your car, lose your spouse or break your arm; you will probably get a stomach ache. Therapy may aim at either desensitizing the organ or stopping the subconscious mind from "shooting" at it. I believe the target organ is often subconsciously selected as symbolically appropriate for some deep emotional or psychological reason.

More conventionally, the term "target organ" refers to the organ innervated by a specific nerve.

Trophic nerve function: This concept does not enjoy wide acceptance. Since 1967, Dr. I.M. Korr has been its leading proponent. The word "trophic" denotes a nutritional function. According to this hypothesis, nerves are essential to the nutrition and consequent growth, development, health and survival of the tissues they serve. It is generally accepted that when a nerve is severed and its end organ shrivels up, it is due to disuse atrophy resulting from the absence of neurotransmitter stimulation of that organ. This is true. But according to the trophic hypothesis, another process is involved: the cell body of a nerve manufactures nutritive protein macromolecules which are delivered by the axon to the end organ. Dr. Korr used radioactive tags of 14C and 32P as tracers to study this delivery system. He reported that sensory end organs are also dependent upon the delivery of nutritive molecules from the cell bodies of their afferent (sensory) nerve cells; i.e., the protein molecules move along the dendrite from the neuron toward the sensory end organ while the electrical wave of stimulation moves in the opposite direction.

Accordingly, the trophic function to a denervated organ must be restored in order to prevent dystrophy. Range of motion exercise alone won't do it. Craniosacral therapy works from the inside out, from the central core to the periphery. Therefore, it may help to reinstitute the flow of proteins along the nerve fibers from the center to the periphery.

The following factors could also interfere with the trophic function of a nerve: a facilitated segment; toxic agents (affecting protein production in the nerve cell body); mechanical tensions involving bones or abnormal myofascial hypertonus (interfering with protein transport along the axon); emotional stress; nutritional problems (affecting protein production and transport); viral infection such as herpes or poliomyelitis; various biochemical problems (e.g., blood acid/alkaline balance) which influence the internal physiological environment.

In my first book (UPLEDGER 1983), I described the physiological rhythm of about 25 cycles per minute found in denervated muscle. Dr. Korr suggests that this change may be due to the loss of trophic function. Since that first writing, I have found this abnormal rhythm in many muscles. After successful treatment, the palpable rhythm has been restored to synchrony with the craniosacral rhythm (10-12 cycles per minute). Partial (as well as total) denervation will cause the 25 cycles per minute rhythm.

Vital life energy: The energy required for life to be present in an animal or plant. Many people now feel that it is electromagnetic in character. There are and have been numerous concepts of vital life energy. The Chinese concept of chi and the Hindu concept of prahna arose many thousands of years ago. More recent Western concepts include the archaeus, liquor vital and Nnmia of Paracelsus; the universal magnetism of

Van Helmont; the life beans of Dr. Robert Fludd; the animal magnetism of Mesmer; the life force of Galvani; the odic force of von Reichenback; the auro as described by Tesla; the N-rays of Blondot; the L-fields of Burr; and the orgone of Reich.

Whiplash: A descriptive term originally applied to the type of injury involving a tissue strain in two directions, much like "cracking a whip." It usually refers to the neck injury resulting from abrupt acceleration or deceleration in an auto accident. In either case, the sudden change in movement of the vehicle causes the victim's head to go in one direction, then in the opposite direction, straining soft tissues on both aspects of the neck.

Recently, this word has been abused such that many people think whiplash means any neck injury except a fracture. Others think it is a legal term meaning there is going to be a lawsuit following the accident. In any case, I'm afraid that whiplash will ultimately join the ranks of such other words as "lumbago," "rheumatism," "the grippe," "migraine" and so on, which have been so overused that they no longer have a valid and precise definition.

REFERENCES

Becker, R.O. 1985. *The Body Electric.* New York: Morrow.

Brain Mind Bulletin. 1985. Vol. 10, Nos. 4/5. Los Angeles.

Chusid, J.G. 1982. *Correlative Neuroanatomy and Functional Neurology.* 18th ed. Los Altos: Lange Medical.

Clemente, C.O., ed. 1985. *Gray's Anatomy.* 30th American ed. Philadelphia: Lea & Febiger.

Costen, J.B. 1936. Neuralgias and Ear Symptoms Associated with Disturbed Function of the Temporomandibular Joint. *J. Amer. Med. Assoc.* 107: 252.

Delacato, C.H. 1963. *The Diagnosis and Treatment of Speech and Reading Problems.* Springfield: Charles C. Thomas.

———— . 1966. *Neurological Organization and Reading.* Springfield: Charles C. Thomas.

Doman, R.G., Delacato, C.H., et. al. 1960. Children with Brain Injuries: Neurological Organization in Terms of Mobility. *J. Amer. Med. Assoc.* 174: 257-262.

Gehin, A. 1985. *Atlas of Manipulative Techniques for the Cranium and Face.* Seattle: Eastland Press.

Harpman, J.A. and Woollard, H.H., 1938. The Tendon of the Lateral Pterygoid Muscle. *J. Anat.* 73: 112.

Hollingshead, W.H. 1968. *Anatomy for Surgeons.* Vol. 1, *The Head and Neck.* p. 97. New York: Harper & Row.

Jones, L.H. 1981. *Strain and Counterstrain.* Colorado Springs: Am. Acad. Osteopathy.

Lavine, R.A. 1983. *Neurophysiology: The Fundamentals.* Lexington: Collarmore.

Netter, F.H. 1983. *The Nervous System.* Vol. 1. West Caldwell: CIBA.

Owman, C. and Edinsson, L., eds. 1977. *Neurogenic Control of Brain Circulation.* pp. 105, 167, 369. New York: Pergamon Press.

Rees, L.A. 1954. Structure and Function of the Temporomandibular Joint. *Brit. Dent. J.* 96: 125.

Restak, R. 1984. *The Brain.* New York: Bantam Books.

Sagan, C. 1977. *Dragons of Eden.* New York: Random House.

Sicher, H. 1944. *Oral Anatomy.* St. Louis: C.V. Mosby.

Sudnow, D. 1978. *Ways of the Hand.* New York: Harper & Row.

Sutherland, W.G. 1967. *Contributions of Thought.* pp. 90-92. Meridian, Idaho: Sutherland Cranial Teaching Foundation.

Upledger, J.E. and Vredevoogd, J.D. 1983. *Craniosacral Therapy.* Chicago: Eastland Press.

Wonder, J. and Donovan, P. 1984. *Whole Brain Thinking.* New York: Morrow.

LIST OF ILLUSTRATIONS

245

INDEX

Items in the following categories are listed under one heading: artery, cartilage, disc, fascia, foramen, fossa, ganglion, gland, ligament, membrane, muscle, nucleus, plexus, sinus, space, tissue, vein. Page numbers for illustrations appear in italics.

N.

O.

P.